GERM CELL

Edited by **Ahmed RG**

Germ Cell
http://dx.doi.org/10.5772/65614
Edited by Ahmed RG

Contributors

Gyeong Hun Baeg, Sharon Wui Sing Tan, Yu Cai, Nicola Bernabò, Luca Valbonetti, Marina Ramal Sancez, Giulia Capacchietti, Mauro Mattioli, Barbara Barboni, Maria P De Miguel, Yago Alcaina, Diego Sainz De La Maza, Alfredo Vitullo, Noelia Leopardo, Pablo Ignacio Felipe Inserra, Pritesh Krishnakumar, Mamta Gupta, Vandana Saini

Published by InTech
Janeza Trdine 9, 51000 Rijeka, Croatia

Publishing Process Manager Edi Lipovic
Technical Editor SPi Global
Cover InTech Design team

First published February, 2018
Printed in Croatia
Legal deposit, Croatia: National and University Library in Zagreb

Additional hard copies can be obtained from orders@intechopen.com

Germ Cell, Edited by Ahmed RG
p. cm.
Print ISBN 978-953-51-3758-0
Online ISBN 978-953-51-3759-7

For EU product safety concerns:
IN TECH d.o.o., Prolaz Marije Krucifikse Kozulić 3, 51000 Rijeka, Croatia,
info@intechopen.com or visit our website at intechopen.com.

Meet the editor

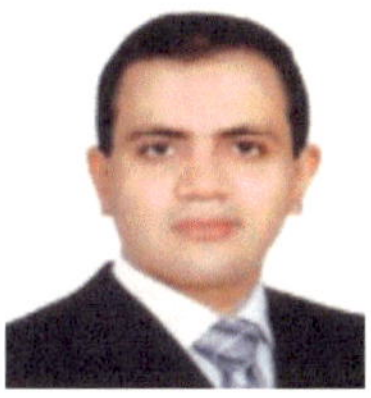

Dr. Ahmed RG received his PhD degree in Developmental Biology (Developmental Endocrinology) from Beni-Suef University, Egypt, and received research training (postdoctoral fellowship) as a visiting scholar at the Catholic University, Belgium. Also, he has outstanding records of scientific and academic accomplishments with multiple research funding, numerous publications (books/papers) in highly prestigious journals, and various presentations in both national and international conferences. He is a member of a number of eminent societies, organizations, and schools. On the other hand, he served as a scientific editor and reviewer for national and international research institutions. He has an honor from Society for Endocrinology in project of You and Your Hormones. He is an assistant director of Animal Housing, Zoology Department, Faculty of Science, Beni-Suef University, Egypt.

Contents

Preface

The book aims to provide an overview of current knowledge regarding germ cells. It deals with the germ cell specification; the regulation of germ line stem cells and their neighboring somatic cells in the fruit fly, *Drosophila melanogaster*; and their reprogramming. In addition, a review is included on the membrane dynamics of spermatozoa during capacitation, new insight into germ cell signaling, and the genotoxic in vitro studies in testicular germ cells. Authors have also contributed articles on the origin, specification, and development of the female germ line in placental mammals and the germ cell tumors and their association with pregnancy. This book will be of interest to scientists, physicians, and lay readers wishing to review recent developments in the field of germ cells.

Ahmed RG
Division of Anatomy and Embryology
Zoology Department
Faculty of Science
Beni-Suef University, Egypt

Chapter 1

Germ Cell Specification: The Evolution of a Recipe to Make Germ Cells

Pritesh Krishnakumar and Roland Dosch

Additional information is available at the end of the chapter

http://dx.doi.org/10.5772/intechopen.71557

Abstract

Multicellular species use gametes for their propagation. Gametes are formed from primordial germ cells (PGCs), which develop during embryogenesis. In some species, PGCs are specified by the inheritance of a RNA granule known as germ plasm. During germ cell specification, the germ plasm conveys a unique set of properties, e.g. the germ cell specific meiotic cell cycle to the PGCs. Germ plasm assembly is controlled by independently evolving organizer proteins like Oskar in *Drosophila* or Bucky ball in zebrafish. These organizers are intrinsically disordered proteins, which rapidly changed their amino acid sequence during evolution. A common recipe has emerged by studies on organizer proteins for animals that use germ plasm to specify their germline. Investigating the nature of these organizers might therefore provide a clue to germ cell specification in other species, which are less accessible to molecular-genetic and embryological approaches. Moreover, we might understand how the first metazoans modified their existing cellular structures from unicellular eukaryotes to ensure their reproduction.

Keywords: zebrafish, germ plasm, primordial germ cell, Bucky ball, Oskar, intrinsically disordered protein, stem cells

1. Introduction

Germ cells are precursors to animal gametes. After fusion, gametes have the impressive capacity to develop into a new organism. As all cells of this organism are descendants of PGCs, they are considered totipotent. Interestingly, gametes are also formed in every subsequent generation from the same germ cell. These features identify germ cells as a truly immortal cell line, whereas somatic cells die at the end of life. These are the same characteristics seen in stem cells, thus making germ cells the superior stem cell.

Germline development has to be tightly regulated and controlled to ensure the development of a fertile adult organism. Any misregulation in the pathway would affect fertility and might lead to no offspring. Eventually, sterility might therefore result in the end of that lineage and ultimately in the extinction of the species. Hence, any errors in the germ cell program could have disastrous consequences for a species compared to mistakes in a somatic cell program like forming an organ.

Compared to somatic tissue, very little is known about the critical period of PGC specification. Understanding the biochemical activity of all germ plasm components could help us to grasp, how germ cells get specified. Furthermore, it could identify how "stemness" is achieved at the molecular level. This knowledge might help to treat many degenerative Wof new drug targets for therapy.

2. Mechanisms of germ cell specification

Two different modes of germ cell specification have been described.

2.1. Inductive mode

Germ cell specification by induction is often described as the ancestral or more prevalent mode (**Figure 1A**) [2]. In the induction mode, germ cell fate is specified through external signals from developing embryonic cells. Induction was described in some invertebrates and in some vertebrates like mammals [3, 4]. The most studied example is the mouse [5–7]. One of the signals inducing germ cells is BMP4 [8]. However, it is currently not clear how conserved this signal is during germ cell specification in other species of the animal kingdom.

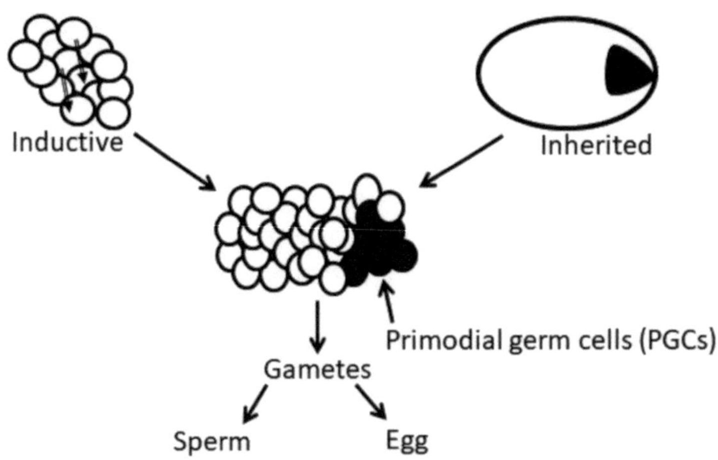

Figure 1. Inherited vs. inductive mode. (A) Inductive mode. Somatic cells induce germ cells (white arrows) within the blastula to express germline factors and differentiate into PGCs (red). (B) Inherited mode. Maternal RNP granules or germ plasm (red) are asymmetrically localized in the oocyte and are inherited by a subset of blastomeres, which specifies PGCs [1].

Regardless whether PGCs are specified by induction or inheritance, they show several commonalities at the molecular level. In most species, numerous proteins and mRNAs like Vasa, Piwi, and Nanos are conserved [9, 10]. In spite of two different modes of specification, they activate common downstream components. We will address the evolutionary conservation of germ plasm again at the end of this chapter, when we describe a potential origin of germ plasm in unicellular organisms.

PGCs adopt different lineages, if transplanted to different parts of the embryo. In the mouse, which uses the induction mode, transplanted PGCs later on colocalize with neural plate and surface ectoderm cells [6]. In *Xenopus*, which uses the inherited mode, transplanted PGCs generate lineages of the three germ layers [11]. These results suggest that despite different specification modes, both types of PGCs still require signaling from extrinsic sources to maintain their fate as fully determined PGCs [12]. Hence, even though the two mechanisms seem starkly different, there may be a common underlying signaling mechanism which is universal.

The key to understanding the specification of PGCs is to separate species-specific adaptations from a core program of germ cell formation. As information about the initial phase of germ cell specification is still quite fragmentary in different organisms, the core program of germ cell specification is unclear. For instance, the molecule that acts as a master or "kick starter" for the germ plasm or PGC program appears to be different in each organism. Therefore, in the rest of this chapter, we will concentrate on the inherited mechanism of germ cell specification.

Publication	Finding/Hypothesis
Weismann (1893)	Inheritance depends on germ cells. Postulates that germ plasm localizes to the nucleus.
Hegner (1911), Boveri (1910)	Germline determinants (germ plasm) localize to the cytoplasm. Germ plasm is necessary (Hegner) and sufficient (Boveri) for germline development.
Bounoure (1934)	Germ plasm for the first time visualized in a vertebrate egg.
Smith (1966)	UV-irradiation of *Drosophila* eggs reduces the number of PGCs. The UV-wavelength suggest that nucleic acids are critical for germline development.
Illmensee and Mahowald (1977)	Ectopic germ plasm is sufficient for PGC formation.
Heasman (1984)	The Balbiani body of *Xenopus* contains the germ plasm.
Ephrussi and Lehman (1992)	Ectopic expression of a single protein termed Oskar gives rise to functional PGCs in *Drosophila*.
Hashimoto (2004)	Ablation of germ plasm in zebrafish reduces PGCs.
Bontems (2009)	Ectopic Expression of a single protein termed Bucky ball induces PGCs in zebrafish.
Brangwynne (2009)	Biophysical studies on embryonic germ plasm reveal a liquid-like hydrogel in *C. elegans*.
Tada (2012)	Germ plasm transplantation in Xenopus induces ectopic germ cells.
Boke (2016)	The *Xenopus* Balbiani body forms amyloid aggregates.

Table 1. Listing selected discoveries that paved the way for the current model of the inherited strategy of germ cell specification.

2.2. Inherited mode

Inheritance of cytoplasmic determinants represents the second mode, by which germ cells are specified (**Figure 1B**). This mechanism of germ cell specification is described amongst others in dipteran insects (e.g. *Drosophila*), nematodes (e.g. *C. elegans*) anuran amphibians (e.g. *Xenopus*), zebrafish, and birds [2, 13]. The molecular mechanisms of germ cell specification are probably better understood at the molecular-genetic and biochemical level than induction, because forward genetics identified most of the known key factors [14, 15]. The best studied examples are probably *Drosophila* and *C. elegans* [16, 17]. **Table 1** summarizes some historical highlights in the context of germ plasm research.

3. Germ plasm

3.1. Composition

Germ plasm is a collection of maternally provided RNAs, proteins, and organelles like mitochondria and endoplasmic reticulum [ER]. The entire assembly forms a cytoplasmic structure in the oocyte named Balbiani body [18]. Sometimes it is also referred to as the mitochondrial cloud in *Xenopus* [19]. The Balbiani body [Bb] was discovered in spiders and it seems to be omnipresent in oocytes of most species of invertebrates (e.g. spiders, insects, and molluscs) and vertebrates (e.g. frogs, birds, teleosts, and mammals) [20–22].

Studies in *Xenopus* and *Drosophila* suggest that the Bb accumulates a subset of mitochondria. These mitochondria are designated to be delivered to the germ plasm and ultimately to the next generation *via* primordial germ cells [23–25]. Interesting experiments in *Drosophila* proposed that germ plasm selects a healthy set of mitochondria by their level of ATP production [23, 24]. The mitochondria in oocytes show high levels of mitochondrial inner membrane potential [26, 27]. Perhaps this mechanism provides germ cells and by extension gametes with the fittest organelles. This ensures that the healthiest mitochondria and its descendants are passed on to the next generation.

3.2. Function

Loss of germ plasm leads to a decrease or no germ cells, whereas in gain of function experiments more germ plasm leads to more germ cells [28] (**Table 1**). Germ plasm components are believed to act in stem cells to convey longevity and totipotency, similar to the magic substances *ambrosia/amrit* in Greek or Hindu mythology, which kept the gods immortal. Many components of germ plasm, like Vasa, are also present in multipotent stem cells flatworms [29]. Nanos is present in stem cells involved in regeneration in planarians [30]. Finally, Piwi also functions in maintaining both germline and somatic stem cells in *Drosophila* [31].

As several germ plasm components have a role in stem cells, it should have a much greater effect in maintaining "stemness" and increased longevity than their somatic stem cell counterparts. As germ plasm conveys a high degree of longevity to germ cells, it would be of stupendous importance to further dissect the germ plasm and study this network of protein and RNA to get further insights into these stemness features.

3.3. Assembly

In the section below, we will concentrate on the two organizer proteins Oskar in invertebrates and Bucky ball in vertebrates that are involved in germ plasm assembly. Both molecules specify germ cells indicating that their biochemistry and mode of action is similar.

4. Oskar in invertebrates

Oskar protein acts as a master regulator of germ plasm assembly [32]. In *Drosophila*, germ plasm is localized to the posterior pole during late oogenesis and hence, also known as pole plasm (**Figure 3**). *Oskar* was isolated in mutagenesis screens for maternal-effect genes required for embryonic patterning [33]. Oskar mutants showed posterior patterning defects and no germ cells [34]. *osk* RNA localizes to the posterior pole, where the protein gets translated and starts the assembly of germ plasm [34, 35]. Mutations in *oskar* affect the enrichment of other RNAs and proteins at the posterior pole, which are present in the germ plasm. This shows that Oskar indeed is essential to initiate germ plasm formation and by extension germ cells.

Mislocalization of Oskar protein at the anterior end of the embryo leads to ectopic germ cells and a second abdomen [32]. Oskar was the first protein, which is both necessary and sufficient to assemble germ plasm. Increasing the amount of Oskar protein in the fly embryo causes an increase in activity of the Nos protein. Thus, the amount of Osk protein and the level of Nos protein accumulation are related. Possibly the heightened expression of Nos represses the somatic cell fate pushing it to a germ cell lineage [36, 37]. Such an activity supports the role of Oskar as a master regulator of PGC specification in invertebrates.

osk mRNA is translated into two protein isoforms by alternative translation initiation [42, 43]. Long Osk (lOsk) is translated at the first start codon and encodes a protein of 606 amino acids. LOsk mainly anchors germ plasm at the posterior end. Long Oskar also traps and accumulates mitochondria at the site of PGC formation. Mutating specifically this long oskar form strongly decreases the number of mtDNA molecules inherited by PGCs [44]. Short Oskar (sOsk) starts at Methionine 139 and encodes a protein of 467 amino acids [42, 43]. sOsk assembles germ plasm and thereby plays a critical role to specify PGCs (**Table 2**).

Long Oskar	Short Oskar
606 amino acids long	467 amino acids long
Anchoring germ plasm	Assembling germ plasm
Associated with endosomes	Associated with RNA granules
Interacts with Lasp to be tethered to posterior pole	Interacts with Lasp to be tethered to posterior pole
Not essential for patterning and germ cell formation	Necessary for germ cell formation and posterior patterning

Table 2. Differences between long and short Oskar.

5. Germ cell specification by Oskar

Fascinating insight into sOsk function was recently gathered by crystallizing two of its domains. These were a domain at the N-terminus of sOsk [139–240aa], which was termed LOTUS domain and previously predicted to be involved in RNA-binding. The second structure described the C-terminal "OSK" domain, which resembles a SGNH hydrolase [40, 41] (**Figure 2**). However, looking carefully at the biochemical interactions and crystallizing sOsk with these binding partners revealed some unexpected information.

sOsk directly interacts with Vasa [45], which is an ATP-dependent helicase [41, 46]. Interesting biochemical and biophysical studies show that the eLOTUS domain of Oskar does not interact with RNA, but in fact binds to the RNA helicase Vasa, which is an important component of germ plasm. Surprisingly, the extension of the LOTUS domain (eLOTUS) encodes an intrinsically disordered motif, which forms a structured domain upon Vasa binding. This stretch of 18 amino acids outside of the LOTUS domain is essential for the Vasa interaction. Moreover, binding the eLOTUS domain increases the ATPase activity of Vasa. This is the first time an instructive role was assigned to Oskar, which was previously regarded as a scaffold protein aggregating germ plasm components within the *Drosophila* oocyte [46].

The OSK domain shows a lot of similarity to a SGNH hydrolase, but lacks three of the four residues of the SGNH motif, as well as the serine triad to be an active hydrolase [41]. The C-terminal OSK-domain forms a globular structure, which carries several basic, positively charged residues at its surface suggesting it could interact with nucleic acids. Indeed, this domain binds in *in vitro* experiments mRNAs like the *osk* and *nos* 3'UTRs [40]. When the basic residues of the OSK domain are mutated, binding to RNA is disrupted [40]. *In vivo* pull-down experiments after UV-crosslinking suggest that Osk interacts with *nos*, *pgc*, and *gcl* mRNA *in vivo* [41]. All three RNAs are known to be localized to the germ plasm. Again, these exciting discoveries identify sOsk as a novel RNA-binding protein and suggest a more instructive role of in germline development than previously anticipated.

Taken the interaction data of sOsk together, a modified picture of germ cell specification emerges. sOsk initiates the assembly of germ plasm by binding to Vasa and mRNA. This interaction activates Vasa and might sterically bring it in proximity with specific RNA(s). This could regulate translation or stability of the RNA(s) involved in specifying PGCs [37]. Hence, Vasa and Osk seem to act in a co-operative manner to specify germ cells.

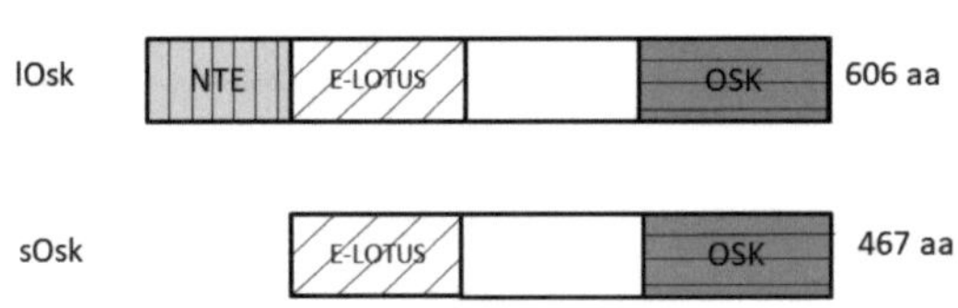

Figure 2. Comparison of long (lOsk) and short (sOsk) Oskar proteins. The NTE domain in lOsk inhibits Vasa-interaction and RNA-binding [16, 38, 39]. The eLOTUS (extended LOTUS) domain consists of the minimal LOTUS domain along with a short disordered region of 18 aa, which together are essential to bind Vasa. The OSK domain binds to RNA [40, 41].

http://dx.doi.org/10.5772/intechopen.71557

Vasa is also involved in piRNA processing. The amount of Vasa in the germ plasm, therefore, prevents the degradation of the germ cell genome by transposon activity, but piRNAs could also play an undiscovered early role in germ cells [47]. Aubergine, a well-known component of the piRNA pathway, is needed for Osk translation, which also needs Vasa to localize. This could indicate a feedback mechanism ensuring all the downstream germ plasm members are expressed [48]. Figuring out the biochemical process, which is initiated by sOsk/Vasa, is probably the key to understand the molecular mechanism of the germ cell specification program.

6. Zebrafish as a model organism to study germ cell specification in vertebrates

Compared to invertebrates such as *Drosophila* and *C. elegans*, much less is known about the molecular processes occurring in the germ plasm of vertebrates. In *Xenopus*, germ plasm research is mostly focused on processes during oogenesis [49–51]. However, among vertebrates that specify their germ cells through inheritance of germ plasm, there are a numerous studies in the zebrafish. Zebrafish combines a number of features helpful for early developmental studies. Embryos and oocytes are easily accessible and available in high numbers. Moreover, its transparent embryos enable tracing of fluorescently tagged proteins *in vivo* and allow detection of endogenous proteins by immunostaining. The genome is completely sequenced, and genomic manipulations via CRISPR/Cas9 are easy. Therefore, zebrafish as a vertebrate model is very well suited for the analysis of germ cell specification [52].

7. Bucky ball in zebrafish

To identify maternal factors controlling early vertebrate development, a maternal-effect mutant screen was carried out in zebrafish [15]. Among the mutants with a defect prior to midblastula transition (MBT), one line produced embryos with radial segregation of cytoplasm instead of animal pole aggregation. In addition, the fertilized embryo from the mutant mother does not show cellular cleavages and hence does not develop beyond the 1-cell stage. As the mutant embryo lacks polarity similar to Buckminsterfullerenes, it was referred to as *bucky ball* (*buc*) [15].

In the oocyte, Buc mutants fail to assemble germ plasm into a Balbiani body (Bb) (**Figure 3A**). Instead, germ plasm components like *nanos* and *vasa* mRNA are no longer localized to the Balbiani body, but rather distributed ubiquitously in the ooplasm [54]. This result described the first gene in vertebrates required for the formation of the Balbiani body and the localization of germ plasm components in the oocyte. Moreover, if the cDNA of Buc is ectopically expressed from a transgene, ectopic Bbs are seen (**Figure 3D**) [55]. This leads to the conclusion that Buc, similar to sOsk in *Drosophila*, is necessary and sufficient for germ plasm assembly.

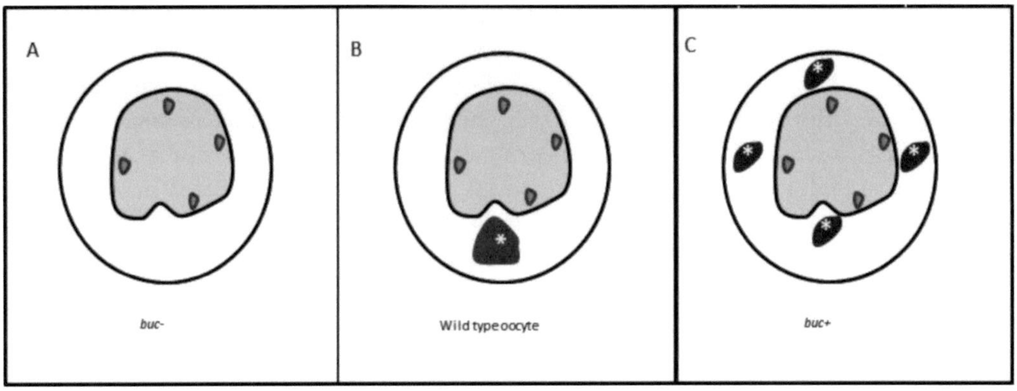

Figure 3. Scheme summarizing the role of Buc for germ plasm assembly during zebrafish oogenesis. (A) In *buc* mutant oocytes *(buc-)*, germ plasm assembly is disrupted, and Balbiani body components are ubiquitously distributed in the oocyte (red haze) [54]. (B) Wild-type stage I zebrafish oocyte, the central nucleus (germinal vesicle; gray), germ plasm/ Balbiani body (red). (C) A transgene with the Buc cDNA is over-expressed, which leads to the ectopic formation of multiple Bbs (red) [54, 55].

7.1. The conservation of Buc across the vertebrate kingdom

Buc is present in vertebrates; however, across its homologs in the vertebrate phylum, the sequence changes quite rapidly [54]. Zebrafish has two paralogs of Buc in its genome, whereas the salmon has three [56]. Currently, the function of the other paralogs is not clear. The *Xenopus* Buc homolog Xvelo exists in two splice forms, long Xvelo and short Xvelo. Both seem to play redudant roles in maintaining germ plasm assembly [51]. In humans, two genetic loci show homology to Buc protein (Gene ID EU128483, EU128484) [54], but the sequence is interrupted by STOP-codons and hence, does not encode an open reading frame. Human ovaries show RNA expression from these loci, but their function is not known (Lyautey et al., unpublished). BUC might act as a noncoding RNA or encode a short peptide [54, 57]. Whether the homologs from other mammals have an open reading frame, like Velo in *Xenopus* or Buc in zebrafish and can in fact induce germ cells, would open an exciting new avenue for stem cell research as well as regenerative medicine.

8. Similarities between Oskar and Buc

Buc and sOsk show a striking homology at the genetic level regarding germ plasm formation. Both mutants show a defect in polarity and a failure of germ plasm aggregation [54, 58]. Remarkably, ectopic overexpression of sOsk and Buc induces the formation of additional germ cells [32, 54]. To this end, no other proteins have been described, which can induce PGC formation in an organism.

Fascinatingly, ectopic expression of *Drosophila* sOsk in zebrafish induces the formation of primordial germ cells similarly to Buc (**Figure 4**) (Krishnakumar et al., unpublished). At the

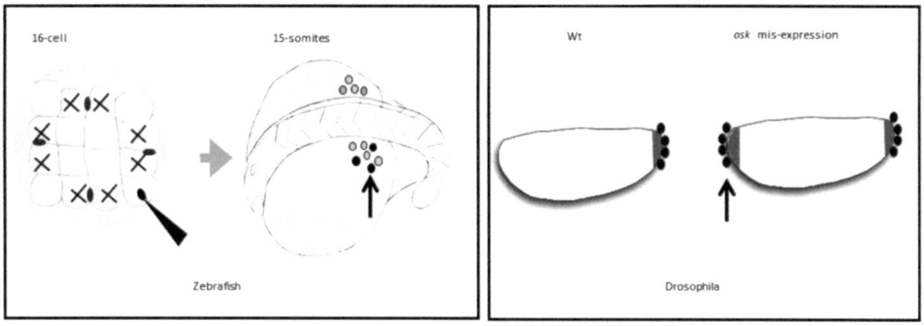

Figure 4. Ectopic PGC induction by germ plasm organizer overexpression. (A) Scheme showing a zebrafish 16-cell embryo in animal view. The middle blastomeres (red) contain endogenous germ plasm and hence, contribute to the PGCs of the embryo. The yellow blastomeres will not participate in germline development and form somatic structures e.g. neurons, muscle, etc. Buc overexpression (green) in a somatic blastomere is sufficient to reprogram germ cells formation. 24hpf stage embryo in a lateral oblique view, anterior to the left. Red cells highlight the endogenous germ cells. Overexpression of Buc in a somatic blastomere leads to the formation of ectopic germ cells (green). (B) Scheme showing *Drosophila* embryos at stage 5, anterior to the left, dorsal to the top. In wt embryos, sOsk is localized to the posterior pole (red), where it induces the formation of ectopic germ cells. Right embryo: germ plasm transplantation or anterior *oskar* localization (red) is sufficient for the specification of ectopic germ cells. Blue arrows point at extra germ cells.

molecular level, *buc* as well as *osk* mRNA localize with other germ cell specific molecules to the germ plasm during oogenesis. This result suggests that Osk and Buc have an overlap in their biochemical network, which they use to form germ plasm and specify germ cells.

sOsk was shown to interact with Vasa, Valois, and Lasp [45, 53, 59]. For example, if Buc also binds to zebrafish Vasa, it could mean that Buc uses a similar set of germ cell core factors like Osk to specify germ cells. *Vice versa,* it would also suggest that Oskar might use zebrafish Vasa to induce germ cells. Taken together, identifying the Buc-interactome might identify conserved factors, which were already core components of the germ cell specification pathway in the first multicellular animals (**Scheme 1**).

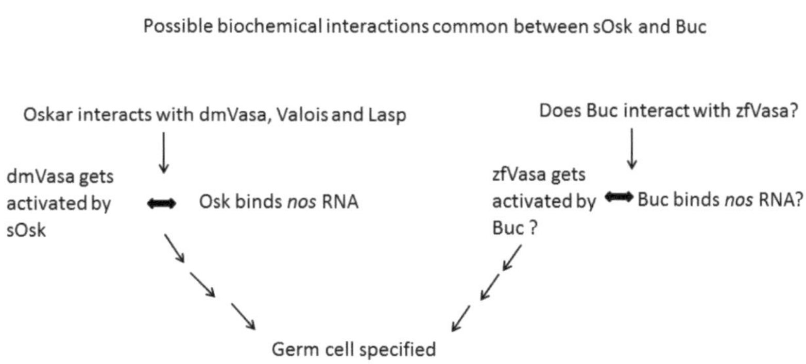

Scheme 1. Osk and Buc could have an overlap in their biochemical network, which they use to form germ plasm and specify germ cells.

8.1. Conservation between Oskar and Buc

According to the sequence-structure-function paradigm, proteins with a conserved activity contain homologous sequence motifs to interact with similar binding partners. Conserved sequences were previously not identified between sOsk and Buc [41, 54, 60]. Buc does not have a visible LOTUS domain, which is required for multimerization and takes part in the interaction with Vasa [46]. Moreover, Buc has no motif with homology to any known RNA binding domain. However, the OSK RNA-binding domain was also not described previously in other proteins and many RNA binding motifs do not show conserved domains [61]. Presently, none of the published bioinformatic analysis detected sequence similarities between the two germ plasm organizers Osk and Buc. Hence, their conserved activity remains a mystery. Overall, this would suggest that the structure or biophysical nature of both proteins might be similar in order to accomplish the same activity by which both would give rise to the "core" RNA-protein complex. sOsk and Buc might, therefore, represent the first protein pair of a frequently postulated phenomenon: Two proteins with similar function without sequence similarity [62].

9. Vasa: the ubiquitous germ cell marker

Vasa seems to be the most widely used molecular marker to identify germ cells [63–67]. Vasa is well conserved during evolution and required for germline development. Vasa is a member of the DEAD-box protein family of RNA helicase suggesting that it resolves duplex RNA or RNA-protein hybrids. Mutations in Vasa show defects in posterior patterning and in germ cell specification in the *Drosophila* embryo [63] . Vasa mutant zebrafish do not form gametes and develop as sterile males [68]. Vasa-null male mice are infertile because their germ cell do not proliferate and differentiate [69]. The VASA-like gene *DBY* in humans also appears to be required for male fertility [70]. In gain of function experiments, ectopic Vasa expression in chicken embryonic stem cells induces expression of specific germline and meiotic genes [71]. When these cells are transplanted into chick embryos, they migrate to the gonad anlagen and differentiate into gametes. Overall these results support the theory that Vasa has a central role in establishing germ line identity and function, however the exact function is still not known.

Vasa RNA or protein expression is frequently used to label PGCs in animals. As at least one homolog seems to be present in all metazoans, Vasa is also an easily accessible marker across the animal kingdom [72]. However, the restriction of Vasa at the blastula stage to the germ plasm and prospective PGCs varies across species. In some species like the zebrafish, Vasa protein is ubiquitous at early stages and later gets restricted into PGCs [73], which raised concerns about the role of Vasa during germ cell specification.

Exciting results from *Drosophila* provided a novel perspective on Vasa and germ cell specification [46]. Vasa has been shown to be activated by sOsk. This would mean that not the localization of Vasa protein or RNA labels the region of the early embryo, where germ cells are specified, but it only matters, where Vasa is active. So far, the activity of Vasa was only determined biochemically by the hydrolysis of ATP, but we still do not know what the activity of Vasa *in vivo* is. It would, therefore, be interesting to differentiate between inactive and active Vasa in the developing embryo and whether the active form labels specified germ cells.

In conclusion, regulatory proteins of Vasa activity like sOsk seem to be a much more reliable marker for germline specification.

10. Low complexity proteins

Low complexity (LC) proteins are of two types, amyloid and intrinsically disordered proteins (IDPs) [74–76]. **Table 3** compares the differences between the two types of LC-proteins.

Both Buc and sOsk have been suggested to have low complexity regions [41, 75, 77]. Indeed, it was shown that sOsk contains an intrinsically disordered region critical for Vasa binding. In Buc and Velo1, it was shown that parts of the conserved BUVE-motif form prions or amyloid-like aggregates. IDPs frequently evolve faster than structured proteins [74, 82]. This feature might hide conserved motifs in both proteins, which are critical to interact with the same biochemical network.

IDPs are also known to act as hubs for supra-molecular complexes and are also more prevalent in RNA-binding proteins. As sOsk fits this profile, it would be interesting to know whether Buc binds RNA to explain their conserved activities. Moreover, IDPs form liquid-liquid phase separations such as RNA-granules, which were also described for the germ plasm in *C. elegans* [79]. Some evidence was provided by *in vivo* imaging of germ plasm in zebrafish [83] and *Drosophila* [84] that germ plasm is liquid. Nonetheless, the level of intrinsic disorder of germ plasm organizers and the liquid properties of germ plasm in fly and fish are still not clear. It is presently unknown how the protein components like Oskar, Vasa, assemble into a germ granule aggregate. RNA-binding proteins have been shown to undergo phase transitions from a soluble to viscous state [85–87]. Thus, RNAs may be trapped by germ plasm aggregates, which become a granule and thereby facilitate more RNA-RNA and RNA-protein interactions. Oskar has been suggested to contain disordered regions, which connect the domains that were crystallized. These regions could push for the propensity to form aggregates as well.

Interestingly, Buc has been discussed to have both amyloid and IDP regions. In *Xenopus*, the Buc homolog Velo1 aggregates into an amyloid like assembly forming the Balbiani body [77].

Properties	Amyloid	IDP
Structure	Low complexity regions form beta sheets.	Very low complexity with FG or FXXG repeats, in most cases with no secondary structure formation.
Chemical	Aggregates are resistant to SDS and high salt concentrations.	Aggregates are dissolved by SDS or high salt concentrations.
Aggregation	Aggregates are resistant to 1,6 hexanediol.	1,6-hexanediol dissolves hydrogels formed by IDPs.
Staining	Stain positively with Thioflavin S and T.	No accumulation of Thioflavin.
	Examples: Amyloid plaques, Balbiani body Xvelo protein in *Xenopus* (Boke et al. [77]).	**Examples**: Nuclear pores [Nucleoporins (Frey et al. [81])], germ plasm in *C. elegans*.

References [77–81].

Table 3. The differences between the two classes of low complexity proteins, amyloid and IDP.

By contrast, BucGFP molecules showed hydrogel or liquid droplet-like behavior in the early zebrafish similar to the P-granules in *C. elegans* [79, 83]. This suggests a controlled transition from an amyloid plaque to a soluble hydrogel at the end of oogenesis. Understanding, how the same protein can generate different aggregates and how these transitions are regulated *in vivo* will be quite exciting. Finding the molecular mechanism, by which the oocyte dissolves amyloids, might also provide a therapeutic strategy to dissolve protein aggregates during neurodegenerative diseases like Alzheimer's.

Overall the aggregation of IDPs emerge as a central theme in germ cell specification. Just like Vasa, which is also intrinsically disordered region [88] and like the polymerizing substrates of P-granules which are the MEG1 and MEG 3 proteins in *C. elegans* [89], Buc and Osk self-aggregate and assemble germ plasm *via* phase transition.

11. A common recipe to make germ cells

If Osk and Buc have diverged from a common ancestor, their precursor would have been an ancient protein of low complexity, which induces germ cell formation. Both proteins probably have unrelated sequences as consequence of their role as intrinsically disordered scaffolds. This structural role releases the constraints to maintain a defined protein structure as described for other IDPs [90]. This divergence probably hides conserved motifs, which bind to a similar interactome such as Vasa, Valois, and probably other common mRNA binding partners (**Figure 5**). Finding interaction partners and mapping the interaction motifs like for the sOsk-Vasa interaction will determine, to which level interaction motifs are conserved between sOsk and Buc.

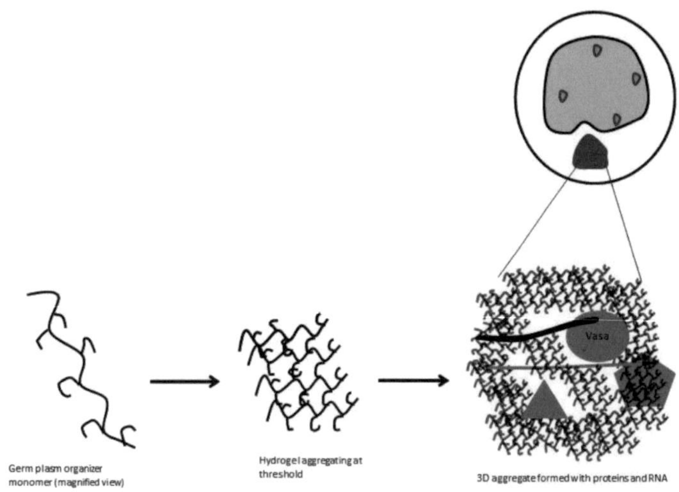

Figure 5. Model for germ plasm formation. Single monomer molecules of germ plasm organizer (red) aggregate through weak interactions of their intrinsically disordered regions (hooks and loops), until a threshold concentration is reached. This leads to a liquid-liquid phase separation (red haze) to form hydrogel-like germ plasm. The aggregate then selectively recruits protein (geometric shapes) and mRNA (lines). This gets packed into germ plasm *e.g.* as shown above in the Balbiani body of the oocyte.

Describing the Balbiani body, a picture of the popular "bubble tea" comes to mind. In this picture, the organizer proteins form a scaffold probably via self-aggregation or upon binding with their interactors similar to the chewy alginate balls, which form during polymerization. During this process, germ plasm assembles and thereby integrates RNA and proteins into this 3D liquid lattice. The assembly also initiates Vasa's activity to start the downstream program, e.g. to protect RNAs and proteins from degradation [91]. The germ plasm also exchanges components with the cytoplasm similar to those spheres floating in the bubble tea. When inherited into a cell, the germ plasm probably releases some proteins whose translation and stability is tightly controlled. Once these factors are unleashed from the bubble spheres, they change the transcriptional program to specify the maturation of a PGC to a gamete.

12. Conclusion

Why should germ cell specification be conserved? Reproduction is a conserved feature of all biological systems and must have been, therefore, be present in the first metazoans before other cell types like neurons, muscle or a vascular system. Germ cell specification was, therefore, present before the formation of an eye or even a nervous system. Nonetheless, the conservation of the master regulator Pax6/Eyeless showed that light sensing organs were already present at the base of metazoan evolution [92]. Although this hallmark finding is currently accepted in the scientific literature, the insect compound eye and the vertebrate camera-eye were regarded as a paradigm for convergent adaptations. We, therefore, speculate that germ cell formation is the more ancient tissue compared to eyes, would use an even more conserved molecular regulation than Pax6/Eyeless.

When animals started to become multi-cellular, they could no longer continue to reproduce by simple cell cleavage. They needed to set the germline apart from the soma for their reproduction [93]. For this task, they had to evolve proteins, which served as master switches for germ cell specification. Any changes to the function of these proteins could have lasting consequences on the propagation of that species. However if these proteins were IDPs, they could still perform their function, despite of rapid (localized or random) changes. These changes could have roles in speciation or better coordinated control of specification. Whatever the case, if they still aggregated and setup the "core" complex, a germ cell would have still formed.

13. Future directions and recommendations: back to the future

Ciliates form a cytoplasmic aggregate called the conjusome [94]. This structure is present only during sexual reproduction. Similar to the Balbiani body in *Xenopus* and the P-granules in *C. elegans*, the conjusome is made up of fibrous, electron dense material [94]. It also contains a Piwi related protein TWI, which protects the integrity of the genome [95]. These commonalities with germ plasm are very striking and suggest that the conjusome might be the ancestral form of germ plasm. Hence, the organizer protein in Ciliates probably displays a very different amino acid sequence from Osk and Buc. However, the Ciliate organizer might have similar characteristics like Osk and Buc, such as forming the protein-RNA core or even induce germ cells in zebrafish. If indeed a germ plasm like structure existed in unicellular organisms, germ cell specification by induction would have emerged after the transition to multicellularity, because signaling requires a multicellular environment. It will, therefore, be quite interesting to find out to which level germ plasm in metazoans and structures like the conjusome in unicellular organisms are conserved. Therefore, if these conjusomes could be chemically isolated, its proteins and RNA can be compared to the known components of germ plasm. This will show if there is an evolutionary clue between the conjusome in lower organisms and germ plasm in higher organisms thus providing the missing link.

Expanding on this hypothesis, protein phase transition might have been present before the first unicellular organisms. If the beginning of life was an RNA world [96] and formation of a cell was needed to protect the genetic material, it would have been easier to have a hydrogel aggregate of slime or protein lock the RNA into an RNA granule than to establish a lipid bilayer with an internal framework. Indeed if that was the case, this structure would have been more similar to the germ plasm that we see today than to a membrane-bound cell. Thus the origin of life would have been from a germ plasm ancestor similar to a drop of Amrit or Ambrosia spilled from the heavens.

Acknowledgements

Pritesh Krishnakumar was supported by the German Academic Exchange Service (DAAD). Research in the Dosch lab is supported by the Deutsche Forschungsgemeinschaft, the GGNB Junior Group Stipend and the "Forschungsförderungsprogramm" of the University Medical Center Goettingen.

Abbreviations

Buc	Bucky ball
Bb	Balbiani Body
C. elegans	*Caenorhabditis elegans*
IDPs	Intrinsically disordered proteins
Osk	Oskar
Pax6	Paired box protein 6
PGCs	Primordial germ cells
RNA	Ribonucleic acid
Xvelo-1	Xenopus Vegetal localized 1

Author details

Pritesh Krishnakumar* and Roland Dosch

*Address all correspondence to: pritesh.krishnakumar@med.uni-goettingen.de

Institute for Developmental Biochemistry, University Medical Center Göttingen, Göttingen, Germany

References

[1] Seervai RNH, Wessel GM. Lessons for inductive germline determination. Molecular Reproduction and Development. 2013;**80**(8)

[2] Extavour CG, Akam M. Mechanisms of germ cell specification across the metazoans: Epigenesis and preformation. Development. 2003;**130**(24):5869-5884

[3] Ullmann SL, Shaw G, Alcorn GT, Renfree MB. Migration of primordial germ cells to the developing gonadal ridges in the tammar wallaby *Macropus eugenii*. Journal of Reproduction and Fertility. 1997;**110**:135-143

[4] Noce T, Okamoto-Ito S, Tsunekawa N. Vasa homolog genes in mammalian germ cell development. Cell Structure and Function. 2001;**26**(3):131-136. Available from: http://www.ncbi.nlm.nih.gov/pubmed/11565805

[5] Toyooka Y, Tsunekawa N, Takahashi Y, Matsui Y. Expression and intracellular localization of mouse vasa-homologue protein during germ cell development. Mechanisms of Development. 2000;**93**:139-149

[6] Tam PP, Zhou SX. The allocation of epiblast cells to ectodermal and germ-line lineages is influenced by the position of the cells in the gastrulating mouse embryo. Developmental Biology. 1996;**178**(1):124-132

[7] Costa Y, Speed RM, Gautier P, Semple CA, Maratou K, Turner JMA, et al. Mouse MAELSTROM: The link between meiotic silencing of unsynapsed chromatin and microRNA pathway? Human Molecular Genetics. 2006;**15**(15):2324-2334

[8] Lawson KA, Dunn NR, Roelen BAJ, Zeinstra LM, Davis AM, Wright CVE, et al. Bmp4 is required for the generation of primordial germ cells in the mouse embryo. 1999;424-436

[9] Seydoux G, Braun RE. Pathway to totipotency: Lessons from germ cells. Cell. 2006;**127**(5): 891-904

[10] Tsuda M. Conserved role of nanos proteins in germ cell development. Science. 2003; **301**(5637):1239-1241. Available from: http://www.sciencemag.org/cgi/doi/10.1126/science.1085222

[11] Tada H, Mochii M, Orii H, Watanabe K. Ectopic formation of primordial germ cells by transplantation of the germ plasm: Direct evidence for germ cell determinant in *Xenopus*.

Developmental Biology. 2012;**371**(1):86-93. Available from: http://dx.doi.org/10.1016/j.ydbio.2012.08.014

[12] Bertocchini F, Chuva de Sousa Lopes SM. Germline development in amniotes: A paradigm shift in primordial germ cell specification. BioEssays. 2016;**38**(8):791-800

[13] Tsunekawa N, Naito M, Sakai Y, Nishida T, Noce T. Isolation of chicken Vasa homolog gene and tracing the origin of primordial germ cells. Development. 2000;**127**(12):2741-2750

[14] Schupbach T, Wieschaus E. Maternal-effect mutations altering the anterior-posterior pattern of the *Drosophila* embryo. Roux's Archives of Developmental Biology: The Official Organ of the EDBO. 1986;**195**(5):302-317

[15] Dosch R, Wagner DS, Mintzer KA, Runke G, Wiemelt AP, Mullins MC. Maternal control of vertebrate development before the midblastula transition: Mutants from the zebrafish I. Developmental Cell. 2004;**6**(6):771-780

[16] Germ LR. Plasm biogenesis—An Oskar-centric perspective. In: Current Topics in Developmental Biology. 1st ed. Vol. 116. Elsevier Inc.; 2016. pp. 679-707. Available from: http://dx.doi.org/10.1016/bs.ctdb.2015.11.024

[17] Strome S, Updike D. Specifying and protecting germ cell fate. Nature Reviews. Molecular Cell Biology. 2015;**16**(7):406-416. Available from: http://www.nature.com/doifinder/10.1038/nrm4009

[18] Kloc M, Jedrzejowska I, Tworzydlo W, Bilinski SM. Balbiani body, nuage and sponge bodies—The germ plasm pathway players. Arthropod Structure & Development. 2014;**43**(4):341-348. Available from: http://dx.doi.org/10.1016/j.asd.2013.12.003

[19] Heasman J, Quarmby J, Wylie CC. The mitochondrial cloud of *Xenopus* oocytes: The source of germinal granule material. Developmental Biology. 1984;**105**(2):458-469

[20] Guraya SS. Recent advances in the morphology, cytochemistry, and function of Balbiani's vitelline body in animal oocytes. International Review of Cytology. 1979;**59**:249-321

[21] von Wittich WH. Dissertatio Sistens Observationes Quaedam de Aranearum ex Ovo Evolutione. Halle, Germany: Halis Saxonum; 1845

[22] Kloc M, Bilinski S, Dougherty MT, Brey EM, Etkin LD. Formation, architecture and polarity of female germline cyst in *Xenopus*. Developmental Biology. 2004;**266**(1):43-61

[23] Cox RT, Spradling ACA. Balbiani body and the fusome mediate mitochondrial inheritance during *Drosophila* oogenesis. Development. 2003;**130**(8):1579-1590

[24] Pepling ME, Spradling AC. Female mouse germ cells form synchronously dividing cysts. Development. 1998;**125**(17):3323-3328

[25] Marinos E, Billett FS. Mitochondrial number, cytochrome oxidase and succinic dehydrogenase activity in *Xenopus laevis* oocytes. Journal of Embryology and Experimental Morphology. 1981;**62**(609):395-409. Available from: http://www.ncbi.nlm.nih.gov/entrez/query.fcgi?cmd=Retrieve&db=PubMed&dopt=Citation&list_uids=6268730

[26] Wilding M, Dale B, Marino M, di Matteo L, Alviggi C, Pisaturo ML, et al. Mitochondrial aggregation patterns and activity in human oocytes and preimplantation embryos. Human Reproduction. 2001;**16**(5):909-917

[27] Tworzydlo W, Kisiel E, Jankowska W, Witwicka A, Bilinski SM. Exclusion of dysfunctional mitochondria from Balbiani body during early oogenesis of *Thermobia*. Cell and Tissue Research. 2016;**366**(1):191-201. Available from: http://dx.doi.org/10.1007/s00441-016-2414-x

[28] Illmensee K, Mahowald AP. Transplantation of posterior polar plasm in *Drosophila*. Induction of germ cells at the anterior pole of the egg. Proceedings of the National Academy of Sciences of the United States of America. 1974;**71**(4):1016-1020

[29] Pfister D, De Mulder K, Hartenstein V, Kuales G, Borgonie G, Marx F, et al. Flatworm stem cells and the germ line: Developmental and evolutionary implications of macvasa expression in *Macrostomum lignano*. Developmental Biology. 2008;**319**(1):146-159

[30] Wang Y, Zayas RM, Guo T, Newmark PA, Nanos Function I. Essential for development and regeneration of planarian germ cells. Proceedings of the National Academy of Sciences of the United States of America. 2007;**104**(14):5901-5906. Available from: http://www.pnas.org/cgi/doi/10.1073/pnas.0609708104

[31] González-Morales N, Géminard C, Lebreton G, Cerezo D, Coutelis JB, Noselli S. The atypical cadherin Dachsous controls left-right asymmetry in *Drosophila*. Developmental Cell. 2015;**33**(6):675-689

[32] Ephrussi A, Lehmann R. Induction of germ cell formation by oskar. Nature. 1992;**358**(6385):387-392. Available from: http://www.nature.com/doifinder/10.1038/358387a0

[33] Lehmann R, Nuesslein-Volhard C. Abdominal segmentation, pole cell formation, and embryonic polarity require the localized activity of oskar, a maternal gene in *Drosophila*. Cell. 1986;**47**(1):141-152

[34] Ephrussi A, Dickinson LK, Lehmann R. Oskar organizes the germ plasm and directs localization of the posterior determinant nanos. Cell. 1991;**66**(1):37-50

[35] Kim-Ha J, Smith JL, Macdonald PM. Oskar mRNA is localized to the posterior pole of the *Drosophila* oocyte. Cell. 1991;**66**(1):23-35

[36] Wang C, Dickinson LK, Lehmann R. Genetics of nanos localization in *Drosophila*. Developmental Dynamics. 1994;**199**:103-115

[37] Smith JL, Wilson JE, Macdonald PM. Overexpression of oskar directs ectopic activation of nanos and presumptive pole cell formation in *Drosophila* embryos. Cell. 1992;**70**(5):849-859

[38] Rongo C, Broihier HT, Moore L, Van Doren M, Forbes A, Lehmann R. Germ plasm assembly and germ cell migration in *Drosophila*. Cold Spring Harbor Symposia on Quantitative Biology. 1997;**62**:1-11

[39] Vanzo NF, Ephrussi A. Oskar anchoring restricts pole plasm formation to the posterior of the *Drosophila* oocyte. Development. 2002;**129**:3705-3714

[40] Yang N, Yu Z, Hu M, Wang M, Lehmann R, Xu R-M. Structure of *Drosophila* Oskar reveals a novel RNA binding protein. Proceedings of the National Academy of Sciences. 2015;**112**(37):11541-11546. Available from: http://www.pnas.org/lookup/doi/10.1073/pnas.1515568112

[41] Jeske M, Bordi M, Glatt S, Müller S, Rybin V, Müller CW, et al. The crystal structure of the *Drosophila* germline inducer Oskar identifies two domains with distinct Vasa helicase- and RNA-binding activities. Cell Reports. 2015;**12**(4):587-598

[42] Markussen F-H, Michon A-M, Breitwieser W, Ephrussi A. Translational control of oskar generates short OSK, the isoform that induces pole plasm assembly. Development. 1995;**3732**(121):3723-3732

[43] Rongo C, Gavis ER, Lehmann R. Localization of Oskar RNA regulates oskar translation and requires Oskar protein. Development. 1995;**121**(9):2737-2746. Available from: http://www.ncbi.nlm.nih.gov/pubmed/7555702

[44] Hurd TR, Herrmann B, Sauerwald J, Sanny J, Grosch M, Lehmann R. Long Oskar controls mitochondrial inheritance in *Drosophila melanogaster*. Developmental Cell. 2016;**39**(5):560-571. Available from: http://dx.doi.org/10.1016/j.devcel.2016.11.004

[45] Breitwieser W, Markussen FH, Horstmann H, Ephrussi A. Oskar protein interaction with vasa represents an essential step in polar granule assembly. Genes & Development. 1996;**10**(17):2179-2188

[46] Jeske M, Müller CW, Ephrussi A. The LOTUS domain is a conserved DEAD-box RNA helicase regulator and essential for recruitment of Vasa to germ plasm. Manuscript submitted Molecular Cell. 2017:939-952

[47] Pek JW, Patil VS, Kai T. piRNA pathway and the potential processing site, the nuage, in the *Drosophila* germline. Development, Growth & Differentiation. 2012;**54**(1):66-77

[48] Harris AN, Macdonald PM. Aubergine encodes a *Drosophila* polar granule component required for pole cell formation and related to eIF2C. Development. 2001;**128**(14):2823-2832

[49] Kosaka K, Kawakami K, Sakamoto H, Inoue K. Spatiotemporal localization of germ plasm RNAs during zebrafish oogenesis. Mechanisms of Development. 2007;**124**(4):279-289

[50] Machado RJ, Moore W, Hames R, Houliston E, Chang P, King ML, et al. *Xenopus* Xpat protein is a major component of germ plasm and may function in its organisation and positioning. Developmental Biology. 2005;**287**(2):289-300

[51] Nijjar S, Woodland HR. Protein interactions in *Xenopus* germ plasm RNP particles. PLoS One. 2013;**8**(11)

[52] Dosch R. Next generation mothers: Maternal control of germline development in zebrafish. Critical Reviews in Biochemistry and Molecular Biology. 2015;**50**(1):54-68. Available from: http://www.tandfonline.com/doi/full/10.3109/10409238.2014.985816

[53] Anne J. Targeting and anchoring Tudor in the pole plasm of the *Drosophila* oocyte. PLoS One. 2010;**5**:e14362

[54] Bontems F, Stein A, Marlow F, Lyautey J, Gupta T, Mullins MC, et al. Bucky ball organizes germ plasm assembly in Zebrafish. Current Biology. 2009;**19**(5):414-422. Available from: http://dx.doi.org/10.1016/j.cub.2009.01.038

[55] Heim AE, Hartung O, Rothhamel S, Ferreira E, Jenny A, Marlow FL. Oocyte polarity requires a Bucky ball-dependent feedback amplification loop. Development. 2014; **141**(4):842-854. Available from: http://dev.biologists.org/cgi/doi/10.1242/dev.090449

[56] Škugor A, Tveiten H, Johnsen H, Andersen Ø. Multiplicity of Buc copies in Atlantic salmon contrasts with loss of the germ cell determinant in primates, rodents and axolotl. BMC Evolutionary Biology. 2016;**16**(1):232. Available from: http://bmcevolbiol.biomedcentral.com/articles/10.1186/s12862-016-0809-7

[57] Chew G-L, Pauli A, Schier AF. Conservation of uORF repressiveness and sequence features in mouse, human and zebrafish. Nature Communications. 2016;**7**(May):11663. Available from: http://www.ncbi.nlm.nih.gov/pubmed/27216465%5Cnhttp://www.pubmedcentral.nih.gov/articlerender.fcgi?artid=PMC4890304

[58] Marlow FL, Mullins MC. Bucky ball functions in Balbiani body assembly and animal-vegetal polarity in the oocyte and follicle cell layer in zebrafish. Developmental Biology. 2008;**321**(1):40-50

[59] Suyama R, Jenny A, Curado S, Pellis-van Berkel W, Ephrussi A. The actin-binding protein Lasp promotes Oskar accumulation at the posterior pole of the *Drosophila* embryo. Development. 2009;**136**(1):95-105

[60] Ahuja A, Extavour CG. Patterns of molecular evolution of the germ line specification gene oskar suggest that a novel domain may contribute to functional divergence in *Drosophila*. Development Genes and Evolution. 2014;**224**(2):65-77

[61] Castello A, Fischer B, Frese CK, Horos R, Alleaume AM, Foehr S, et al. Comprehensive identification of RNA-binding domains in human cells. Molecular Cell. 2016;**63**(4):696-710. Available from: http://dx.doi.org/10.1016/j.molcel.2016.06.029

[62] Doolittle RF. Similar amino acid sequences: chance or common ancestry? Science. 1981; **214**(4517):149-159

[63] Lasko PF, Ashburner M. The product of the *Drosophila* gene vasa is very similar to eukaryotic initiation factor-4A. Nature. 1988;**335**:611-617

[64] Raz E. The function and regulation of vasa-like genes in germ-cell development Erez Raz. Genome Biology. 2000;**1**(3):1-6

[65] Lasko PF, Ashburner M. Posterior localization of vasa protein correlates with, but is not sufficient for, pole cell development. Genes & Development. 1990;**4**:905-921

[66] Yajima M, Wessel GM. Essential elements for translation: The germline factor vasa functions broadly in somatic cells. Development. 2015;**142**:1960-1970

[67] Tomancak P, Guichet A, Zavorszky P, Ephrussi A. Oocyte polarity depends on regulation of gurken by Vasa. Development. 1998;**125**:1723-1732

[68] Hartung O, Forbes MM, Marlow FL. Zebrafish vasa is required for germ-cell differentiation and maintenance. Molecular Reproduction and Development. 2014;**81**(10):946-961

[69] Ikenishi K, Tanaka TS. Spatio-temporal expression of *Xenopus* Vasa homolog, XVLG1, in oocytes and embryos: The presence of XVLG1 RNA in somatic cells as well as germline cells. Development, Growth & Differentiation. 2000;**42**(2):95-103

[70] Foresta C, Ferlin A, Moro E. Deletion and expression analysis of AZFa genes on the human Y chromosome revealed a major role for DBY in male infertility. Human Molecular Genetics. 2000;**9**(8):1161-1169

[71] Lavial F, Acloque H, Bachelard E, Nieto MA, Samarut J, Pain B. Ectopic expression of Cvh (Chicken Vasa homologue) mediates the reprogramming of chicken embryonic stem cells to a germ cell fate. Developmental Biology. 2009;**330**(1):73-82

[72] Van Doren M, Broihier HT, Moore LA, Lehmann R. HMG-CoA reductase guides migrating primordial germ cells. Nature. 1998;**396**(6710):466-469

[73] Knaut H, Pelegri F, Bohmann K, Schwarz H, Nüsslein-Volhard C. Zebrafish vasa RNA but not its protein is a component of the germ plasm and segregates asymmetrically before germline specification. The Journal of Cell Biology. 2000;**149**(4):875-888

[74] Dyson HJ, Wright PE. Intrinsically unstructured proteins and their functions. Nature Reviews. Molecular Cell Biology. 2005;**6**(3):197-208

[75] Toretsky JA, Wright PE. Assemblages: Functional units formed by cellular phase separation. The Journal of Cell Biology. 2014;**206**(5):579-588

[76] Oldfield CJ, Dunker AK. Intrinsically disordered proteins and intrinsically disordered protein regions. Annual Review of Biochemistry. 2014;**83**:553-584. Available from: http://www.ncbi.nlm.nih.gov/pubmed/24606139

[77] Boke E, Ruer M, Wühr M, Coughlin M, Lemaitre R, Gygi SP, et al. Amyloid-like self-assembly of a cellular compartment. Cell. 2016;**166**(3):637-650

[78] Kroschwald S, Maharana S, Mateju D, Malinovska L, Nüske E, Poser I, et al. Promiscuous interactions and protein disaggregases determine the material state of stress-inducible RNP granules. eLife. 2015;**4**(August):1-32

[79] Brangwynne CP, Eckmann CR, Courson DS, Rybarska A, Hoege C, Gharakhani J, et al. Germline P granules are liquid droplets that localize by controlled dissolution/condensation. Science. 2009;**324**(5935):1729-1732. Available from: http://www.sciencemag.org/cgi/doi/10.1126/science.1172046

[80] Coletta A, Pinney JW, Solís DYW, Marsh J, Pettifer SR, Attwood TK. Low-complexity regions within protein sequences have position-dependent roles. BMC Systems Biology. 2010;**4**(1):43. Available from: http://www.biomedcentral.com/1752-0509/4/43

[81] Frey S, Richter RP, Gorlich D. FG-rich repeats of nuclear pore proteins form a three-dimensional meshwork with hydrogel-like properties. Science. 2006;**314**(5800):815-817. Available from: http://www.sciencemag.org/cgi/doi/10.1126/science.1132516

[82] Malinovska L, Kroschwald S, Alberti S. Protein disorder, prion propensities, and self-organizing macromolecular collectives. Biochimica et Biophysica Acta, Proteins and Proteomics. 2013;**1834**(5):918-931. Available from: http://dx.doi.org/10.1016/j.bbapap.2013.01.003

[83] Riemer S, Bontems F, Krishnakumar P, Gömann J, Dosch RA. Functional Bucky ball-GFP transgene visualizes germ plasm in living zebrafish. Gene Expression Patterns. 2015;**18**(1-2):44-52. Available from: http://dx.doi.org/10.1016/j.gep.2015.05.003

[84] Sinsimer KS, Lee JJ, Thiberge SY, Gavis ER. Germ plasm anchoring is a dynamic state that requires persistent trafficking. Cell Reports. 2013;**5**(5):1169-1177. Available from: http://dx.doi.org/10.1016/j.celrep.2013.10.045

[85] Brangwynne CP. Phase transitions and size scaling of membrane-less organelles. The Journal of Cell Biology. 2013;**203**(6):875-881

[86] Lin Y, Protter DSW, Rosen MK, Parker R. Formation and maturation of phase-separated liquid droplets by RNA-binding proteins. Molecular Cell. 2015;**60**(2):208-219. Available from: http://dx.doi.org/10.1016/j.molcel.2015.08.018

[87] Zhang Y, Cao H, Liu Z. Binding cavities and druggability of intrinsically disordered proteins. Protein Science. 2015;**24**(5):688-705

[88] Nott TJ, Petsalaki E, Farber P, Jervis D, Fussner E, Plochowietz A, et al. Phase transition of a disordered nuage protein generates environmentally responsive membraneless organelles. Molecular Cell. 2015;**57**(5)

[89] Wang JT, Smith J, Chen BC, Schmidt H, Rasoloson D, Paix A, et al. Regulation of RNA granule dynamics by phosphorylation of serine-rich, intrinsically disordered proteins in *C. elegans*. eLife. 2014;**3**:1-23

[90] Forman-Kay JD, Mittag T. From sequence and forces to structure, function, and evolution of intrinsically disordered proteins. Structure. 2013;**21**(9):1492-1499. Available from: http://dx.doi.org/10.1016/j.str.2013.08.001

[91] Aguero T, Kassmer S, Alberio R, Johnson A, King ML. Vertebrate Development. Vol. 9532017. pp. 383-440. Available from: http://link.springer.com/10.1007/978-3-319-46095-6

[92] Gehring WJ. New perspectives on eye development and the evolution of eyes and photoreceptors. The Journal of Heredity. 2005;**96**(3):171-184

[93] Grosberg RK, Strathmann RR. The evolution of multicellularity: A minor major transition? Annual Review of Ecology, Evolution, and Systematics. 2007;**38**(August):621-654. Available from: http://ecolsys.annualreviews.org

[94] Janetopoulos C, Cole E, Smothers JF, Allis CD, Aufderheide KJ. The conjusome: A novel structure in Tetrahymena found only during sexual reorganization. 1999;**1011**:1003-1011

[95] Mochizuki K, Fine NA, Fujisawa T, Gorovsky MA. Analysis of a piwi-related gene implicates small RNAs in genome rearrangement in Tetrahymena. 2002;**110**:689-699

[96] Cech TR. The RNA world in context. RNA Worlds. 2010:9-13

Chapter 2

The Regulation of Germline Stem Cells and Their Neighbouring Somatic Cells in the Fruit Fly (*Drosophila melanogaster*)

Sharon Wui Sing Tan, Yu Cai and Gyeong Hun Baeg

Additional information is available at the end of the chapter

http://dx.doi.org/10.5772/intechopen.69963

Abstract

The *Drosophila* germline stem cells (GSCs) remain as one of the most well-understood adult stem cells. The number of stem cells that self-renews and differentiates must be tightly controlled to maintain tissue homeostasis. The *Drosophila* GSCs are maintained by local signals emanated from the niche, which is composed of the surrounding somatic cells. Notably, GSC homeostasis is also known to be influenced by systemic signals and external stimuli. The *Drosophila* hormone ecdysone and its signalling cascade were found to regulate GSC homeostasis. The insulin signalling pathway as well as nutrient availability can also regulate GSC number. Furthermore, neuronal sex peptide signalling induced in female flies after mating was shown to increase GSC number. Hence, the *Drosophila* GSC system serves as a useful model towards understanding the mammalian stem cells. Compared with the mammalian stem cell models, the *Drosophila* GSC system is anatomically simpler where stem cells can be easily identified, imaged and manipulated genetically. Nevertheless, recent findings have facilitated our understanding into how GSCs and their neighbouring somatic cells sense and respond to changes in a variety of local, systemic and external stimuli.

Keywords: *Drosophila*, germline stem cells (GSCs), stem cell niche, nutrients, insulin signalling, insulin-like peptides (Ilps), ecdysone, sex peptide (SP), mating

1. Introduction

Germline stem cells (GSCs) are adult stem cells that give rise to gametes. Sperm and egg production is an important process, whereby genetic information is transferred to the next generation by GSCs. Hence, GSC self-renewal and differentiation must be tightly regulated to ensure a homeostasis for a healthy egg and sperm production. The GSCs in both female and male *Drosophila* are one of the best-understood adult stem cells by far. The *Drosophila* is a useful in vivo model to study how GSCs and their surrounding somatic cells are co-regulated. Short-range signals from GSC niche, systemic signals and external stimuli aid to determine the fate of GSCs. Upon these signals, GSCs undergo asymmetric divisions, whereby they self-renew to produce one cell that remains as a stem cell and another daughter cell that is displaced away from the niche and is fated to differentiate. The daughter cell maintains its stemness because it stays in direct contact to and receives immediate signals from the niche, whereas the other daughter cell receives low/no signals because it is further away from the niche and, hence, is programmed to differentiate. Under certain circumstances such as genetic mutation or impaired internal or external signals, GSCs become poorly regulated, leading to over-proliferation of GSCs (GSC tumours) or precocious differentiation of the GSCs (GSC loss). Both conditions are unfavourable for the organism as they can cause infertility and hence impaired reproduction and endangering the species population. In this chapter, a brief description on the *Drosophila*'s ovary and testis will be covered. In addition, the molecular mechanisms underlying GSC maintenance by short-range signals produced from the niche and long-range signals such as hormones and insulin-like peptides produced from the brain or external stimuli such as nutrient availability and mating will be discussed.

2. The *Drosophila* ovary and testis germ cell system

2.1. The *Drosophila* ovary system

The female *Drosophila* has a pair of ovaries each of which consists of about 17 repeated units called the ovarioles. The ovarioles are further subdivided into two main parts with the anterior region being the germarium, and a series of gradually differentiated egg chambers are positioned at the posterior end. The germarium is where all the stem cell activity takes place, and there are two types of stem cells present in the germarium: GSCs which eventually generate gametes and somatic stem cells (SSCs, also referred to as follicle stem cells (FSCs)). The apical tip of the germarium consists of approximately 8–10 terminal filament (TF) cells followed by 5–7 cap cells (CCs) at the base of TF cells which are directly in contact with 2–3 GSCs [1–3]. The cap, TF cells and ECs (escort cells that line at the surface of the anterior half of the germarium) provide the stem cell niche for the regulation of GSCs by short-range signals. The GSCs divide asymmetrically to produce one daughter cell that stays in contact with the CCs and hence maintains its stem cell identity and another daughter cell that moves away from the niche to differentiate called a cystoblast (CB) [4, 5]. Loss of GSCs can signal the neighbouring GSCs to go through symmetric division, producing two daughter cells that both retain GSC fate and stay in contact with CCs; hence, this mechanism replaces the unoccupied niche space [6]. The GSCs stay connected to the CCs through adherens junction and loss of *adherens junction* can lead to GSCs moving away from the niche to differentiate [7]. GSCs and its differentiated progeny can be recognized by the presence of fusome, which are germ-specific organelles rich in membrane skeletal proteins like the α-spectrin and hu-li tai shao (Hts) [8, 9]. The fusome appears round in shape (also referred to as spectrosome) in GSCs and cystoblasts (CBs) but is branched in the CB progenies. In the female, the fusome degenerates shortly after the formation of 16-cell cysts [8]. The CBs will undergo synchronous division with incomplete cytokinesis to produce 2-, 4-, 8- and 16-cell cysts. The early cyst cells are encased by long cytoplasmic extension from escort cells (ECs), whereas the late-stage cysts are encased by follicle cells (FCs) produced by the FSCs [10]. The 16-cell cysts surrounded by FCs will bud off from the germarium to produce individual egg chambers [10]. The female GSCs are dominantly regulated by the bone morphogenic protein (BMP) signalling from the niche. In *Drosophila*, the *decapentaplegic* (*dpp*) and *glass-bottom boat* (*gbb*) are ligands for BMP and are mainly expressed in the TF cells and CCs. Loss of *dpp* and *gbb* caused GSCs to dive into differentiation mode, whereas too much of *dpp* leads to over-proliferation of GSCs and forms GSC tumours [11, 12]. The *bag of marbles* (*bam*) and *benign gonial cell neoplasm* (*bgcn*) are essential for CB differentiation [13–15]. CBs lost the ability to differentiate with *bam* loss of function and eventually form germline tumour [11, 14]. On the other hand, overexpression of *bam* caused loss of GSCs as seen in *dpp* loss of function [11, 16]. BMP signalling promotes GSC self-renewal by the mechanism, whereby mothers against *dpp* (Mad) is phosphorylated leading to the formation of Mad and Med complex, which subsequently translocates into the nucleus to bind to *bam* promoter and, hence, represses the transcription of *bam* in GSCs [12]. The GSC niche formed by TF cells, CCs and ECs also expresses P-element-induced wimpy testis (*piwi*), *fs*(1)*Yb* (also known as *Yb*) and *hedgehog* (*hh*), which are required for GSC maintenance [17–19]. *Piwi* and *hh* expressions in the GSC niche require *Yb*. Loss of function of *piwi* and *Yb* in the GSC niche causes GSC exhaustion as seen in *BMP* signalling mutants, whereas overexpression of *piwi* or *Yb* expands GSC number to 2.5-folds, although the increase was not as dramatic as *dpp* overexpression which led to GSC tumour [17, 19]. *Hh* mutation in the GSCs niche affects the GSC population at a lower rate which may suggest that it has a minor role in GSC maintenance [19]. Additionally, Hh signalling activation in ECs promotes germline differentiation [20–22]. Besides that, the Notch signalling controls the formation of GSC niche, whereby elevated *Notch* signalling resulted in increased niche size (CC number) and hence more GSCs; reduced *Notch* signalling resulted in decreased CC number and niche size which in turn reduced the number of GSCs (**Figure 1**) [23].

2.2. The *Drosophila* testis system

The male *Drosophila* has a pair of testes and at the apical tip is where the stem cell niche is housed. The stem cell niche consists of postmitotic hub cells, GSCs and cyst stem cells (CySCs). In the male *Drosophila*, about 6–12 GSCs are arranged in a rosette pattern around a tightly packed cluster of hub cells by adherens junction rich in E-cadherin [24, 25]. Each GSC is encased by a pair of somatic CySCs, which are also in contact with the hub cells by their cytoplasmic extensions such that the distance of the CySC nuclei is further from the hub cells compared to the GSC nuclei [26]. The female and male GSCs have many processes in common; one of them is the asymmetric division of GSCs to produce one daughter cell that self-renews and another that differentiates. By doing so, the male GSCs generate one daughter cell that stays in contact with the hub cells and retains its stem cell identity and another daughter cell that is further away from the hub cells, called gonialblast (GB). The GB is fated for differentiation due to the lack of local signals it receives from the

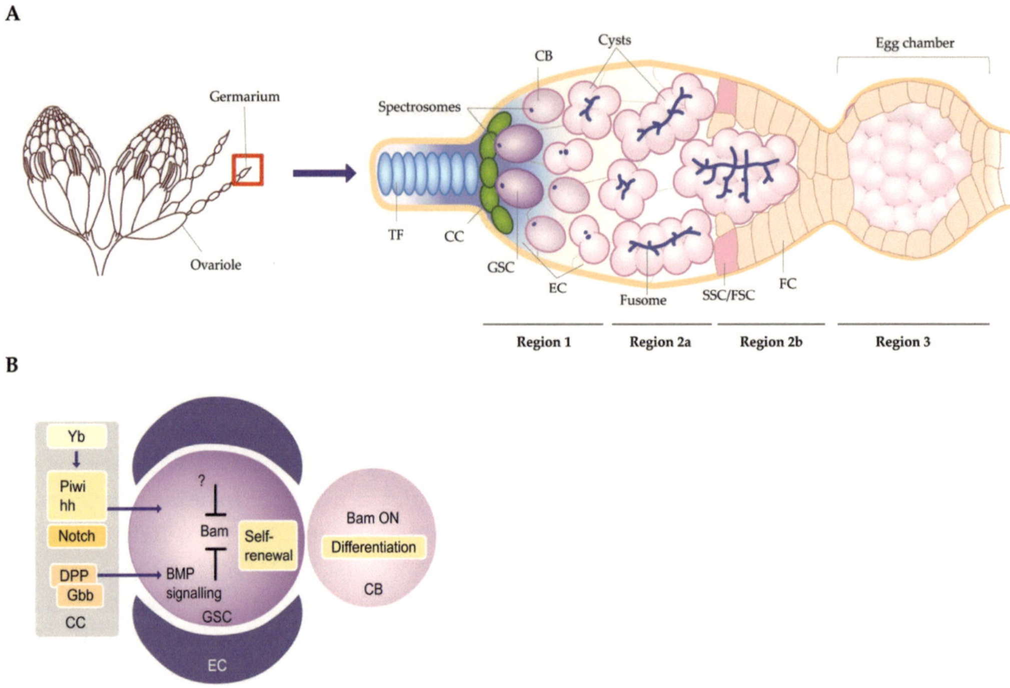

Figure 1. A schematic diagram of the *Drosophila* ovary. (**A**) A pair of *Drosophila* ovaries consisting of several ovarioles each and the zoom in section of the germarium. (**B**) The stem niche of the *Drosophila* ovary consisting of TF, CC and GSC and the signalling pathways that maintain the niche.

niche and is programmed to advance into four rounds of transit-amplifying divisions to generate 2-, 4-, 8- and 16-spermatogonial cells. These 16-spermatogonial cells will then enter the premeiotic S-phase followed by spermatocyte growth and spermatogenesis to produce spermatids and eventually mature sperms [27]. A pair of cyst cells which are progenies of CySCs continue to completely wrap around each GB and its progenies of differentiated spermatogonial cells; cyst cells do not increase in number but only grow to accommodate the expanding spermatogonial cells. CySCs and cyst cells provide protective layer which also isolate germ cells from each other, and only ring canals can connect the spermatogonial cells together [27]. The spectrosomes also appear spherical in the GSCs and GBs but are branched fusome in the differentiated spermatogonial cells. However, unlike the fusome in the ovaries which perishes after mitosis, fusome in the *Drosophila* testis continues to develop further through meiosis and spermatid elongation [28].

The male GSCs are also regulated by local signals from the niche to ensure a balanced population of germ cells. The Janus kinase-signal transducers and activators of transcription (JAK-STAT) signalling pathway was the first to be discovered to regulate GSCs in the fly testis. The ligand of the pathway called *Unpaired* (*Upd*) is expressed in the hub cells, whereby it activates the JAK-STAT signalling in the adjacent GSCs and CySCs. When the transcription factor STAT is exhausted from the testis, GSCs and CySCs are lost, whereas misexpression of *Upd* led to GSCs and CySCs that can self-renew without close proximity to the niche [29, 30]. Activation of *STAT* in somatic cells outside the niche is adequate to initiate CySC and GSC self-renewal but, *STAT* activation in GSCs was inadequate to activate GSC self-renewal outside the niche. This suggests that

CySCs with activated JAK-STAT signalling may provide signals which support the self-renewal of adjacent GSCs and that CySC loss might have directly caused the loss of GSCs in the previous *STAT* depletion study [31]. The zinc-finger homeodomain protein 1 (zfh1) is expressed in the CySCs and is required for its maintenance. Zfh1 is a target of JAK-STAT, whereby it is likely that the activation of BMP ligands in the CySCs is through zfh1 [31]. The expression of *zfh1* in the cyst cells outside the niche caused self-renewal of CySCs and GSCs outside the niche as seen in previous similar study with *STAT* [32]. Chronologically inappropriate morphogenesis (chinmo) is another target of JAK-STAT signalling, and it is required for CySC maintenance [33]. Just like in the female *Drosophila*, the BMP signalling is likewise involved in the regulation of GSCs in the *Drosophila* testis. *Dpp* and *gbb* are expressed in both the hub cells and CySCs, and they activate the self-renewal of GSCs while repressing the transcription of *bam* (**Figure 2**) [34–37].

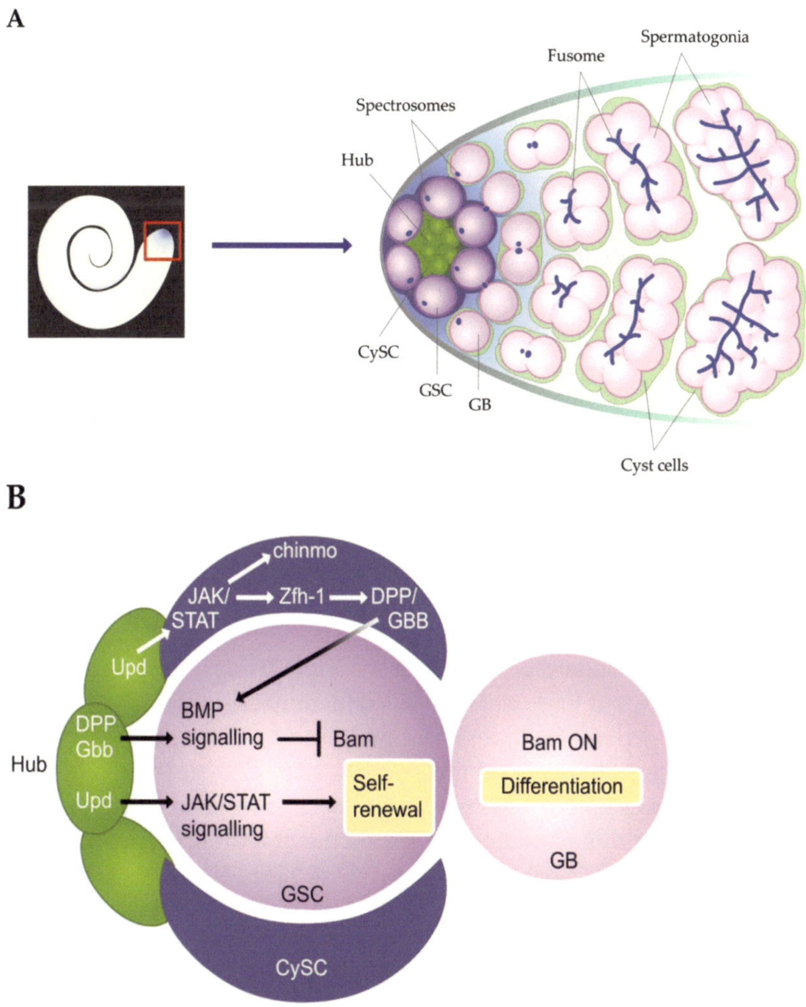

Figure 2. A schematic diagram of the *Drosophila* testis. (**A**) A *Drosophila* testis and the zoom in section of the apical tip of the testis. (**B**) The stem niche of the *Drosophila* testis consisting of the Hub, GSC and CySC and the signalling pathways that maintain the niche.

3. Nutrients and the insulin signalling pathway regulate the germ cell system in both the ovary and testis of *Drosophila*

3.1. Nutrition plays a big role in the development of *Drosophila* ovary

Besides the local signals from the niche, stem cells can respond to external signals such as changes in nutrient availability. Under life-threatening environment such as starvation, organisms often respond by compromising their developmental and/or reproductive programmes. When female flies were fed with diet lacking protein (poor diet), egg-laying was greatly affected with 60-fold difference compared to flies fed on a yeast-rich diet. The ovaries were also greatly reduced in size under poor diet. These effects can be seen within 1 day of switching the flies from normal to poor food, and it takes 2 days for these flies to recover from the effect of poor food to normal egg production and ovary size. Such rapid reproductive changes suggest that egg production is highly dependent on changes in nutrition. Switching female flies from normal to poor food caused a reduction in proliferation rates in both germline and somatic stem cells as well as their progenies to two to fourfold. This is to a lesser extent when compared to female flies raised entirely on poor diet. Although the proliferation rates were reduced, the number of active stem cells remained the same. On the other hand, a checkpoint mechanism was identified at the region 2a and 2b of the germarium. Under poor nutrient condition, apoptosis of the cyst cells was detected at the region where FCs first begin to surround the germline cysts. Cysts moving through the 2a region are preparing for meiosis, and nutrient limitation might have activated cell death programme of both the cysts and somatic cells. Lacking somatic cells to envelope the cysts, this programmed cell death upon nutrient deprivation can prevent insufficient somatic cells from encasing the cyst and cause developmental lapse. The dramatic decline in egg production under poor nutrition might have been due to a slower proliferation programme of the germ line and FSCs and its progenies as well as apoptosis that occurred in the 2a and 2b region [38].

3.2. Nutrition regulates GSCs and CySCs in the *Drosophila* testis

Just like the female flies, the male germ cells are also affected by poor nutrition. When male flies were switched from standard food to poor food for 20 days, their testes become much thinner overtime. The GSCs of these testes declined in numbers to about 35% and nearly 50% for CySCs and early cyst cells. The number of proliferating GSCs measured by cells in the S-phase of mitotic division also reduced greatly from 28 to 17% on 20 days of poor diet. No apoptosis of germ cells was detected in starving flies suggesting that apoptosis did not cause the loss of GSCs but direct differentiation. As seen in the fly ovaries, such phenotypes caused by nutrient deprivation are reversible. Upon switching flies back to normal diet after poor diet, testis development improved, and their testes returned to normal size. The proliferation of GSCs resumed leading to healthy GSC number, and spermatogonia repopulated the testis tip [39]. The ovaries and testes of the flies prove to be not the only organs affected by poor nutrition. The fly intestinal stem cells (ISCs) and its daughter cell called the enteroblast (EB) showed the same effect. The intestine became much smaller, and both the ISCs and EB reduced in numbers when switched from rich to poor diet. When rich food was available again after starving, the intestine regained its original size. ISCs proliferated at a normal rate, and both ISCs and EB increased in numbers [39].

3.3. The insulin signalling pathway as the nutrient sensor which regulates the development of *Drosophila* ovary

The *Drosophila* insulin signalling pathway has been known for its role in regulating the body, organ and cell size of the animal as well as ageing and lifespan. In *Drosophila*, the insulin signalling consists of insulin-like peptides (Ilps), insulin receptor (InR) and insulin-like substrate or chico which are mediated by the PI3K, phosphoinositide-dependent kinase 1 (Pdk1) and Akt pathway. Genetic defects in components of the pathway caused developmental delays in *Drosophila* giving rise to smaller body and cell size, less cells, increased fat and sterile females. These effects are not caused by insulin signalling alone but can be seen in flies that were starved during development which suggests a link between the insulin signalling pathway and nutrient availability [40, 41]. In fact, research done on the endoreplicating tissues (ERTs) which constitute majority of the *Drosophila* larva showed that inhibition of *PI3K* can suppress cell growth as seen in starved animal; introducing *InR* or *PI3K* can rescue cell loss in starved animal; and *PI3K* activity is activated when nutrition is available [41].

There are seven *Drosophila* insulin-like peptides (Ilps) in total with three (*Ilp2, Ilp3 and Ilp5*) being produced in two clusters of the medial neurosecretory cells in both larvae and adult *Drosophila* brain [42, 43]. However, among the three Ilps produced in the brain, only *Ilp3* and *Ilp5* are regulated by nutrient availability, whereas *Ilp2* remain stable during starvation. The Ilp5 is also found in the FCs of the female adult ovaries [44]. The remaining *Ilps* are expressed in other parts of the animal such as imaginal discs, gut and ventral nerve cord [43]. When neurosecretory cells were ablated in the third instar larvae, female adult flies which eclosed later on showed a severe reduction in ovary size and vitellogenic oocytes leading to decreased fecundity [44]. The ability of FCs to proliferate was severely affected in female flies with ablated neurosecretory cells even when rich food was available [45]. A partial decline in proliferation of follicle cells can likewise be seen in female flies with homozygous mutation for *chico* and fed on rich food, reminiscence of flies on poor food. *Chico* mutant caused a serious impairment of egg chambers to develop beyond vitellogenesis in spite of the availability of rich food [38]. Besides that, loss of neurosecretory cells can cause a reduction in body weight and wing area of eclosed flies and reduced length of larvae to half the normal size, and development was slowed down by double [44, 46]. The developmental delays caused by fewer neurosecretory cells can be rescued by expression of *Ilp2* during larvae stage but not the proliferation rate of the FCs [45]. These larvae also have higher levels of glucose and trehalose compared to wild type, and this can be rescued when *Ilp2* was expressed which suggests that insulin signalling pathway can regulate energy metabolism in the animal [46]. Unlike in mammals where Ilps are produced in the pancreas, expression of Ilps in the brain is common in insects [47–49]. For instance, the *Bombyx mori* secretes Ilps from the neurosecretory cells in response to nutrients [50]. Taken together, this shows that the brain is the main organ that produces Ilps to control oogenesis, development and energy metabolism.

When the *Drosophila insulin receptor* (*InR*) was mutated in the germ cells of female flies, the development and size of the germline cysts were greatly reduced. Germ cells with homozygous mutant for *InR* led to cysts which fail to complete vitellogenesis and degenerate. A complete loss of function of *InR* in the germ line resulted in a comprehensive hindrance in vitellogenesis. However, such hindrance was only partial when the neurosecretory cells were ablated. Therefore, Ilp5 produced in the follicle cells most likely works together with the brain Ilps to control vitellogenesis. On the other hand, *InR* mutation in the GSCs of the female flies divides at a much slower rate, and their division rate is dependent on *InR* activity, suggesting that GSCs receive Ilp signal directly and not through the niche to regulate its division [45]. There were less GSCs and CCs in *InR* mutant compared to control, and such loss of GSCs and CCs was quicker with increased age which can be suppressed by overexpression of *Ilp2* in somatic cells. CCs with *InR* mutation showed decreased ability to attach to GSCs due to changes in E-cadherin levels [51]. Loss of *chico* in the female GSCs caused a decline in GSCs and its division rate which can be rescued when wild-type *chico* transgene was introduced or *PI3K* was activated in the GSCs [45, 51].

3.4. The insulin signalling pathway regulates the GSCs in *Drosophila* testis

In the male flies, the *InR* is expressed in the hub cells, GSCs and early germline and somatic cells. Loss of GSCs was seen when *InR* mutation was activated for 10 days in the GSCs. Constitutive expression of *InR* in early germ cells resulted in partial rescue of GSC loss in starved flies, whereas expression of *InR* in both the GSCs and hub cells led to a significant suppression of GSC loss. Similar trend was seen when the activated form of *Drosophila PI3K* was expressed in both the GSCs and hub cells. These results indicate that *InR* can regulate GSC maintenance and constitutive activation of *InR* in the GSCs and hub cells can effectively overturn the loss of GSCs under poor nutrition [39]. A combination of *InR* mutation can cause sterility in both male and female flies. In male sterile flies, their testis showed a reduction of germ cells or sperms. Further investigations showed a decrease in GSCs with increased age in these *InR* mutant male flies. A severe decrease in spermatocyte cysts was also found in testes with *InR* or *chico* mutation even in newly eclosed males. Ablation of neurosecretory cells can also cause a decline in spermatocyte cysts. *InR* mutant testes also showed a decrease in phosphorylated Akt compared to control suggesting that loss of GSCs and spermatocyte cysts can be caused by inactive insulin signalling through the PI3K/Akt pathway. Besides that, *InR* mutation in the testes affected the cell cycle progression of GSCs. There were less GSCs in the S-phase and G2/M phase of the mitotic cycle in the *InR* mutant testes. The spermatocytes undergo a dramatic increase in size before meiosis takes place. These results suggest that InR plays a role in the asymmetric division of the male GSCs, the cell cycle progression of GSCs and the cell growth of spermatocytes [52]. The CySCs of the male *Drosophila* requires the PI3K/target of rapamycin (Tor) activity to differentiate, and lack of which directs the CySCs into a proliferative state [53].

In another study, centrosome misorientation was found to be the culprit of GSC loss or GSC proliferation delay caused by reduced insulin signalling or poor nutrition in male flies. The cell cycle of GSCs is halted in the event of centrosome misorientation and will resume once the orientation is back to normal [54–56]. Male flies under poor nutrition had higher percentage of GSCs with misoriented centrosome compared with flies grown on rich food. However, the spindle orientation remained normal which advocates that the centrosome orientation checkpoint was intact. This means that the GSCs had a slower cycling rate under poor nutrition. The impaired centrosome orientation was reversible and restored within 3–5 days when flies under poor diet were transferred to rich diet. To investigate if centrosome misorientation can be affected by insulin signalling, a dominant-negative form of *InR* or hypomorphic *InR* mutant was expressed in the germ cells, and the result was a significant increase in centrosome misorientation occurrence regardless of nutrient condition. When the active form of *InR* was expressed, centrosome misorientation reduced significantly even in poor diet. Another component of the insulin signalling pathway, Akt, also regulates centrosome orientation. Knockdown of *Akt* led to high frequency of centrosome misorientation, and the opposite effect can be seen in overexpression of *Akt* regardless of nutrient condition. Overexpression of *Ilp1, Ilp2, Ilp3, Ilp5* and *Ilp6* also reduced centrosome misorientation even in poor food, but this effect was not seen in *Ilp4* and *Ilp7* overexpression. These suggest that GSC centrosome orientation or GSC proliferation is controlled by insulin signalling pathway and nutrient availability (**Figure 3**) [57].

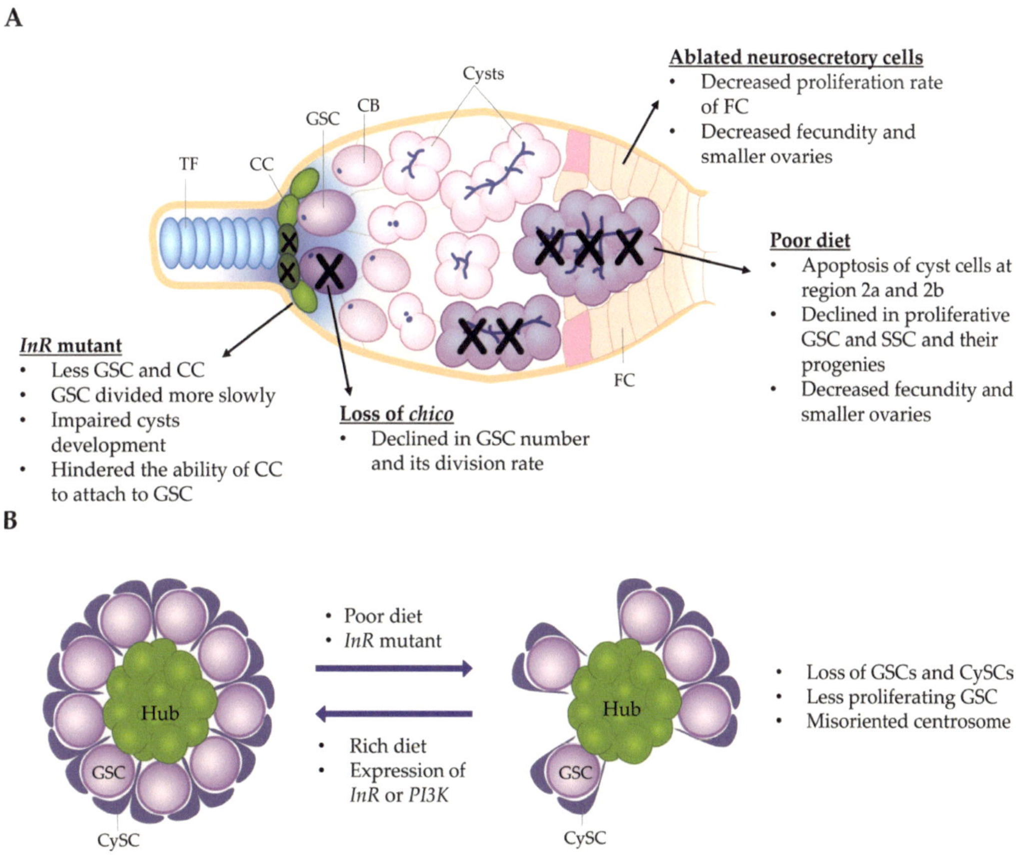

Figure 3. The effect of nutrient availability and insulin signalling pathway on the *Drosophila* ovary and testis. (**A**) A summary of the effect of poor diet and disrupted insulin signals on the *Drosophila* ovary. (**B**) The effect of poor diet and compromised insulin signalling pathway on the stem cell niche of the *Drosophila* testis and such effects are reversible when conditions become favourable again.

4. Steroid signalling regulates the development of *Drosophila* ovary and testis

The endocrine system plays a role in development, metamorphosis, oogenesis and stem cell maintenance in *Drosophila* [58–60]. The major steroid hormone in *Drosophila* is ecdysteroids or its active form, twenty-hydroxyecdysone (20E) which is analogous to the human sex steroids [61]. The 20E acts by binding to a heterodimeric nuclear receptor complex which comprises of an ecdysone receptor (EcR) and ultraspiracle (Usp). EcR and usp have mammalian orthologues, franesoid X receptor/liver X receptor and retinoid X receptor, respectively [62, 63]. The 20E/EcR/Usp complex will then bind to the ecdysone response elements (EcREs) to activate transcription or repression of various genes [64–66]. The early response genes of ecdysone signalling consist of E74, E75 and Broad-Complex (BR-C) which all play a role in egg chamber development [67, 68]. The ecdysteroids were first discovered in the ovaries of adult mosquitoes and subsequently found to be expressed in the ovaries of adult *Drosophila* [69–72]. *EcR* null mutation caused very few female flies (approximately 2% of females) to lay eggs, and they stop laying eggs at day 4–5, suggesting the requirement of ecdysone signalling for oogenesis. Besides, the enzyme important for steroid hormone synthesis was also found to regulate egg chamber development. When *dare,* the *Drosophila* homologue for the enzyme *adrenodoxin reductase,* was mutated, fewer female flies laid eggs, and they progressively lost their ability to lay eggs [67].

Mutation in the biosynthesis of ecdysone or *EcR* encourages GSCs to progress through G2 phase of cell cycle which showed increase in G2/M fusomes. However, these mutations also caused a rapid loss in GSC number. The ecdysone early response gene *E74* but not others was found to regulate GSCs as well. When mutated, GSCs showed significant decline in their division rate. There was also a surge in apoptopic cysts and decline in late-stage cysts which were not seen in *usp* inactivation and may suggest that *E74* is required for the survival of cysts. This seems to be similar to what was found in insulin signalling which also promotes GSC progression through G2 phase. However, E74 acts independently of insulin signalling because removal of a downstream target of insulin signalling, forkhead box, subgroup O (FOXO) has no effect in division of *E74* mutant GSCs [73]. The chromatin remodelling factor called imitation SWI (ISWI) was known to be involved in the self-renewal of *Drosophila* ovary GSCs [74]. This study found ecdysone signalling to work together with ISWI-containing nucleosome remodelling factor (NURF) complex to regulate GSCs in the *Drosophila* ovary. There was an amplified loss in GSCs in combined mutation of *nurf301* and *EcR, ISWI* and *EcR* and *ISWI* and *E74*. The BMP signalling was also regulated by ecdysone, whereby phosphorylated Mad (pMad), which is the downstream effector of BMP signalling, was decreased in *usp* and *E74* mutation GSCs. A decline or loss in GSCs was also seen in combined mutation of *EcR* and *dpp,* a BMP ligand [73]. These results show that steroid hormones can alter the epigenetic status of stem cells to influence their fate as well as affecting their capability to receive signals from the niche.

Another finding showed that downregulation of *taiman* (a steroid receptor co-activator) in ECs increased the number of GSCs and CCs and disruption of ecdysone signalling or the biosynthesis of ecdysone caused excessive germ cells with single spectrosome [75]. In another study, mutation in the biosynthesis of ecdysone and knockdown of *usp*, *EcR* or the response gene, *E75*, in the somatic cells can all affect early oogenesis, whereby regions 1 and 2a of the germarium became significantly reduced in size. Mutation in ecdysone and its signalling in the germarium also caused a rapid loss in GSC number as well as reduced 16-cell cysts. Besides that, depleted ecdysone signalling caused severe impairment in the development of new 16-cell cyst and entry into meiosis [76].

The male *Drosophila* is known to have lower titers of 20E as compared to the females. Nevertheless, the hormone is present in the *Drosophila* testis, and the ecdysone signalling is also required for stem cell maintenance. Male flies deprived of ecdysone caused by mutation led to far less GSCs. Mutation in *EcR* caused significant loss of CySCs and GSCs with 8-cell spermatogonia detected right next to the hub. Besides that, knocking down *EcR* or *usp* specifically in the CySCs and its lineages resulted in a significant decline in CySCs as well as GSCs. This may suggest that *EcR* and *usp* are required nonautonomously in CySCs for GSC maintenance. Interestingly, expression of *EcR-B2* (an isoform of *EcR*) in the CySC lineage can rescue the loss of both stem cell populations seen earlier in *EcR* mutation [77].

5. Mating acts as an external stimulus that regulates GSC number in the *Drosophila* ovary

Another external stimulus that can affect GSC number is mating. During mating, the male-derived sex peptide (SP) is received by the sex peptide receptor (SPR), which is expressed in the female genital tract and its nervous system [78, 79]. Female flies that mated had more GSCs compared to the virgin females, and such increase in GSCs lasted for only 6 days, consistent with the period that sperm can sustain upon mating. There was no increase in GSC number when female flies mated with male flies depleted of *SP* or in female flies with loss of *SPR* function, suggesting the involvement of SP signalling in regulating mating-induced GSC number. Expression of *SP* gene in the neurons of virgin females resulted in increase of GSC number, but such effect was not detected when the somatic cells of the ovaries were overexpressed with *SP* [80]. Another study showed that mating caused a surge in the level of ecdysteroid in *Drosophila* ovaries and, hence, the steroid hormone regulated the mating-induced increase in GSCs [80]. The sensory neurons in the female uterus and oviduct expressed neuronal markers like *fruitless* (*fru*) and *pickpocket* (*ppk*). Disrupting the synaptic transmission of these neurons impersonated the presence of *SP* and caused virgin female flies to become less receptive to mating and stimulated egg-laying. These might suggest that activation of *SPR* by *SP* reduced the synaptic transmission of the sensory neurons. It was also established that the neuronal signal initiated by the *SP* is delivered to the central nervous system [79]. These suggest that mating acts as an external stimulus which sends signal to the sensory neurons in the female genital tract to the central circuits which then alter the female reproductive behaviour leading to more egg production to ensure the survival of the species (**Figure 4**).

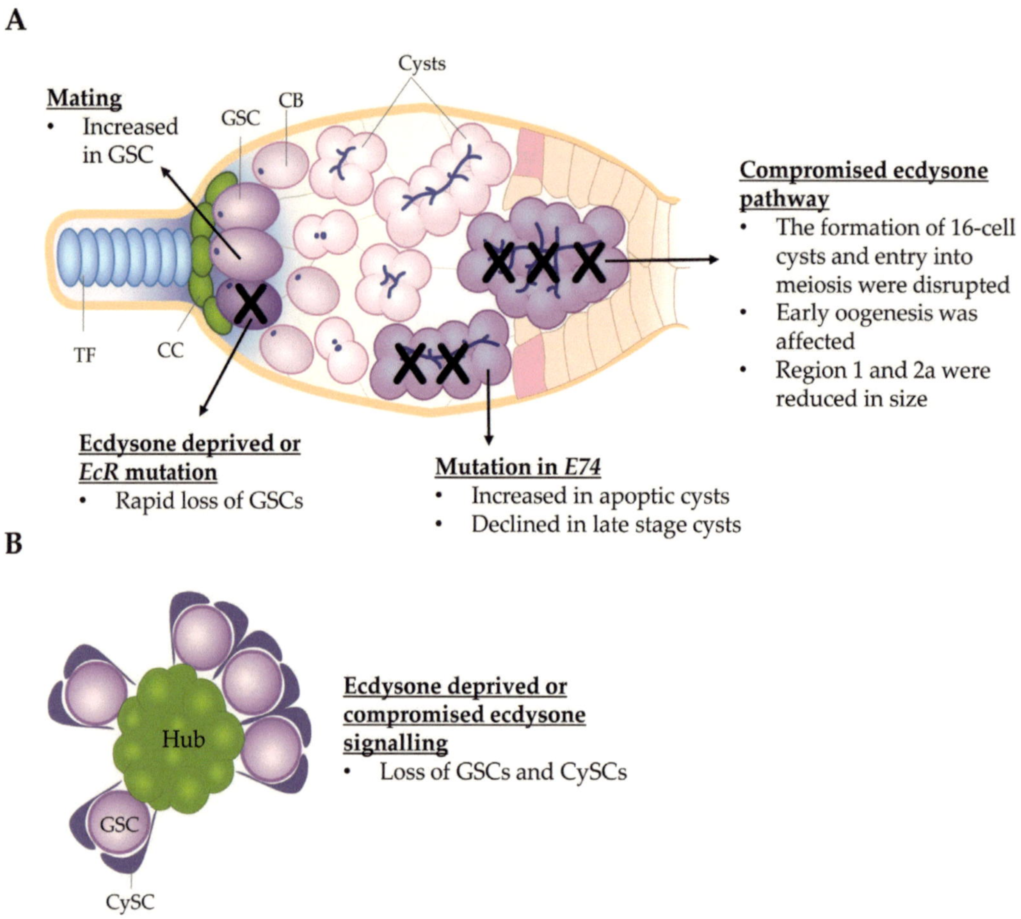

Figure 4. The effect of the ecdysone hormone and its signalling pathway on the *Drosophila* ovary and testis. (**A**) A summary of the effect of mating, deprived ecdysone and its disrupted signalling pathway on the *Drosophila* ovary. (**B**) Hormone deprivation and its compromised signalling pathway can affect the GSC and CySC number of the *Drosophila* testis.

6. Conclusion

The germline stem cell system in both female and male *Drosophila* has been advantageous in providing a platform to address fundamental questions in stem cell biology. As many features of the *Drosophila* stem cell biology are conserved, the studies done on *Drosophila* can have an extensive implication on our understanding of the mammalian stem cell system and, hence, aid in the development of regenerative medicine. The recent work on the *Drosophila* ovaries and testes has shed light on our general understanding of stem cell behaviour. It has revealed the complex regulatory network of the stem cell niche that constantly maintains GSCs, which then develop progressively to give rise to functional gametes when required. Moreover, it is remarkable to see how the brain is involved in safeguarding an organ or cells that are so far apart from itself. Not only does the brain produce insulin-like peptides that regulate germ cells, but mating can also send signals to the brain to induce egg production in germline or amend the reproductive behaviour in the females. Besides that, the stem cell niche proved to be resilient and flexible at the same time, whereby they can sense and respond to internal and external changes as described above. It is also worth to note that compromised internal or external changes very often just reduced the number of GSCs and the surrounding somatic cells or caused them to divide more slowly instead of going through severe programmed cell death. It is as though nature has its way to preserve these GSCs in bad times and is definitely better to have less functional GSCs than to have none. Besides that, in times when conditions become favourable again, the very few GSCs left can repopulate the lost GSCs by symmetric division or turning on or off specific signalling pathway to quickly get back on track. Given the requirement of GSCs to pass on the genome to its future generation, this is definitely an intelligent way to ensure that the species is being preserved.

7. Future directions

The *Drosophila* ovary and testis stem cell niches are a complex system to a certain extent; however, more insights can be gained through various genome-wide assays such as large-scale RNAi screening or gene expression profiling to identify new players whose loss of function either enhance or inhibit stem cell self-renewal. Ongoing and future studies will persist to disclose the complex network of signalling pathways that control the maintenance of GSC and the adjacent somatic cells and how these signalling pathways function and respond to changes in their external and internal environment. The somatic cells that surround the germ cells have not received enough attention despite their importance in maintaining the germ cells. It would be interesting to reveal how the two different cell populations exchange signals from each other, especially under unfavourable conditions. Besides that, it has been known that the GSCs in both the female and male *Drosophila* can be replenished through mechanisms such as dedifferentiation of differentiated germ cells or via symmetric division of the GSCs. However, what drives such phenomena to occur remains largely unexplored. Since poor nutrition or unfavourable hormone signalling can cause loss of GSCs, will these GSCs be replenished after prolong exposure to unfavourable external or internal environment and would it be through dedifferentiation or symmetric division? In addition, although both the ovary and testis systems are very similar in many aspects, there are still obvious differences between the two. For example, there are multiple stem cell niches present in the ovary due to the presence of several ovarioles compared to only one stem cell niche in the *Drosophila* testis. Furthermore, there might be more distinct mechanisms underlying GSC maintenance which are present in one system but not the other. There are endless interesting questions to be explored and will take many more years of research for us to fully understand these complex systems. Most importantly, the studies done on the *Drosophila* ovary and testis will help us understand adult stem cells and design therapeutic interventions for stem cell-related disorders in a whole new level.

Abbreviations

20E	Twenty-hydroxyecdysone
bam	Bag of marbles
bgcn	Benign gonial cell neoplasm
BMP	Bone morphogenetic protein
BR-C	Broad-Complex
CC	Cap cell
CB	Cystoblast
CySC	Cyst stem cell
dpp	*Decapentaplegic*
E74	Ecdysone-induced protein 74EF
E75	Ecdysone-induced protein 75B
EB	Enteroblast
EC	Escort cell
EcR	Ecdysone receptor
EcRE	Ecdysone response element
ERT	Endoreplicating tissue
FC	Follicle cell
FOXO	Forkhead box, subgroup O
FSC	Follicle stem cell
fru	Fruitless
GB	Gonialblast
gbb	Glass-bottom boat
GSC	Germline stem cell
Hh	Hedgehog
Hts	Hu-li tai shao
InR	Insulin receptor
Ilp	Insulin-like peptide
ISC	Intestinal stem cell
ISWI	Imitation SWI
JAK-STAT	Janus kinase-signal transducers and activators of transcription
Mad	Mothers against *dpp*
NURF	Nucleosome remodelling factor
Pdk1	Phosphoinositide-dependent kinase 1
Piwi	P-Element-induced wimpy testis
pMad	Phosphorylated Mad
Ppk	Pickpocket
SP	Sex peptide
SPR	Sex peptide receptor
SSC	Somatic stem cell
TF	Terminal filament
Tor	Target of rapamycin

http://dx.doi.org/10.5772/intechopen.69963

Upd	Unpaired
Usp	Ultraspiracle
Yb	Female sterile (1) Yb
Zfh1	Zn-finger homeodomain protein 1

Acknowledgements

This was supported by MOE AcRF Tier 1 grant (R-181-000178-112) to BGH. The authors would like to thank Ms. Song-Lin Bay for her assistance in preparing the artwork for the figures used in this chapter.

Author details

Sharon Wui Sing Tan[1], Yu Cai[2,3] and Gyeong Hun Baeg[1]*

*Address all correspondence to: antbgh@nus.edu.sg

1 Department of Anatomy, Yong Loo Lin School of Medicine, National University of Singapore, Singapore

2 Temasek Life Sciences Laboratory, National University of Singapore, Singapore

3 Department of Biological Sciences, National University of Singapore, Singapore

References

[1] Decotto E, Spradling AC. The *Drosophila* ovarian and testis stem cell niches: Similar somatic stem cells and signals. Developmental Cell. 2005;**9**(4):501-510

[2] Wieschaus E, Szabad J. The development and function of the female germ line in *Drosophila melanogaster*: A cell lineage study. Developmental Biology. 1979;**68**(1):29-46

[3] Lin H, Spradling AC. Germline stem cell division and egg chamber development in transplanted *Drosophila* germaria. Developmental Biology. 1993;**159**(1):140-152

[4] Lin H, Spradling AC. A novel group of pumilio mutations affects the asymmetric division of germline stem cells in the *Drosophila* ovary. Development. 1997;**124**(12):2463-2476

[5] Deng W, Lin H. Spectrosomes and fusomes anchor mitotic spindles during asymmetric germ cell divisions and facilitate the formation of a polarized microtubule array for oocyte specification in *Drosophila*. Developmental Biology. 1997;**189**(1):79-94

[6] Xie T, Spradling AC. A niche maintaining germ line stem cells in the *Drosophila* ovary. Science. 2000;**290**(5490):328-330

[7] Song X, Zhu CH, Doan C, Xie T. Germline stem cells anchored by adherens junctions in the *Drosophila* ovary niches. Science. 2002;**296**(5574):1855-1857

[8] Lin H, Yue L, Spradling AC. The *Drosophila* fusome, a germline-specific organelle, contains membrane skeletal proteins and functions in cyst formation. Development. 1994;**120**(4):947-956

[9] de Cuevas M, Lee JK, Spradling AC. alpha-spectrin is required for germline cell division and differentiation in the *Drosophila* ovary. Development. 1996;**122**(12):3959-3968

[10] Margolis J, Spradling A. Identification and behavior of epithelial stem cells in the *Drosophila* ovary. Development. 1995;**121**(11):3797-3807

[11] Xie T, Spradling AC. *decapentaplegic* is essential for the maintenance and division of germline stem cells in the *Drosophila* ovary. Cell. 1998;**94**(2):251-260

[12] Song X, Wong MD, Kawase E, Xi R, Ding BC, McCarthy JJ, et al. Bmp signals from niche cells directly repress transcription of a differentiation-promoting gene, bag of marbles, in germline stem cells in the *Drosophila* ovary. Development. 2004;**131**(6):1353-1364

[13] McKearin DM, Spradling AC. bag-of-marbles: A *Drosophila* gene required to initiate both male and female gametogenesis. Genes & Development. 1990;**4**(12B):2242-2251

[14] McKearin D, Ohlstein B. A role for the *Drosophila* bag-of-marbles protein in the differentiation of cystoblasts from germline stem cells. Development. 1995;**121**(9):2937-2947

[15] Lavoie CA, Ohlstein B, McKearin DM. Localization and function of Bam protein require the benign gonial cell neoplasm gene product. Developmental Biology. 1999;**212**(2):405-413

[16] Ohlstein B, McKearin D. Ectopic expression of the *Drosophila* Bam protein eliminates oogenic germline stem cells. Development. 1997;**124**(18):3651-3662

[17] Cox DN, Chao A, Lin H. piwi encodes a nucleoplasmic factor whose activity modulates the number and division rate of germline stem cells. Development. 2000;**127**(3):503-514

[18] King FJ, Lin H. Somatic signaling mediated by fs(1)Yb is essential for germline stem cell maintenance during *Drosophila* oogenesis. Development. 1999;**126**(9):1833-1844

[19] King FJ, Szakmary A, Cox DN, Lin H. Yb modulates the divisions of both germline and somatic stem cells through piwi- and hh-mediated mechanisms in the *Drosophila* ovary. Molecular Cell. 2001;**7**(3):497-508

[20] Li C, Kan L, Chen Y, Zheng X, Li W, Zhang W, et al. Ci antagonizes Hippo signaling in the somatic cells of the ovary to drive germline stem cell differentiation. Cell Research. 2015;**25**(10):1152-1170

[21] Lu T, Wang S, Gao Y, Mao Y, Yang Z, Liu L, et al. COP9-Hedgehog axis regulates the function of the germline stem cell progeny differentiation niche in the *Drosophila* ovary. Development. 2015;**142**(24):4242-4252

[22] Liu Z, Zhong G, Chai PC, Luo L, Liu S, Yang Y, et al. Coordinated niche-associated signals promote germline homeostasis in the *Drosophila* ovary. The Journal of Cell Biology. 2015;**211**(2):469-484

[23] Song X, Call GB, Kirilly D, Xie T. Notch signaling controls germline stem cell niche formation in the *Drosophila* ovary. Development. 2007;**134**(6):1071-1080

[24] Spradling A, Fuller MT, Braun RE, Yoshida S. Germline stem cells. Cold Spring Harbor Perspectives in Biology. 2011;**3**(11):a002642

[25] Fuller MT, Spradling AC. Male and female *Drosophila* germline stem cells: Two versions of immortality. Science. 2007;**316**(5823):402-404

[26] Hardy RW, Tokuyasu KT, Lindsley DL, Garavito M. The germinal proliferation center in the testis of *Drosophila melanogaster*. Journal of Ultrastructure Research. 1979;**69**(2):180-190

[27] de Cuevas M, Matunis EL. The stem cell niche: Lessons from the *Drosophila* testis. Development. 2011;**138**(14):2861-2869

[28] Hime GR, Brill JA, Fuller MT. Assembly of ring canals in the male germ line from structural components of the contractile ring. Journal of Cell Science. 1996;**109**(Pt 12):2779-2788

[29] Tulina N, Matunis E. Control of stem cell self-renewal in *Drosophila* spermatogenesis by JAK-STAT signaling. Science. 2001;**294**(5551):2546-2549

[30] Kiger AA, Jones DL, Schulz C, Rogers MB, Fuller MT. Stem cell self-renewal specified by JAK-STAT activation in response to a support cell cue. Science. 2001;**294**(5551):2542-2545

[31] Leatherman JL, Dinardo S. Germline self-renewal requires cyst stem cells and stat regulates niche adhesion in *Drosophila* testes. Nature Cell Biology. 2010;**12**(8):806-811

[32] Leatherman JL, Dinardo S. Zfh-1 controls somatic stem cell self-renewal in the *Drosophila* testis and nonautonomously influences germline stem cell self-renewal. Cell Stem Cell. 2008;**3**(1):44-54

[33] Flaherty MS, Salis P, Evans CJ, Ekas LA, Marouf A, Zavadil J, et al. chinmo is a functional effector of the JAK/STAT pathway that regulates eye development, tumor formation, and stem cell self-renewal in *Drosophila*. Developmental Cell. 2010;**18**(4):556-568

[34] Shivdasani AA, Ingham PW. Regulation of stem cell maintenance and transit amplifying cell proliferation by tgf-beta signaling in *Drosophila* spermatogenesis. Current Biology. 2003;**13**(23):2065-2072

[35] Kawase E, Wong MD, Ding BC, Xie T. Gbb/Bmp signaling is essential for maintaining germline stem cells and for repressing bam transcription in the *Drosophila* testis. Development. 2004;**131**(6):1365-1375

[36] Schulz C, Kiger AA, Tazuke SI, Yamashita YM, Pantalena-Filho LC, Jones DL, et al. A misexpression screen reveals effects of bag-of-marbles and TGF beta class signaling on the *Drosophila* male germ-line stem cell lineage. Genetics. 2004;**167**(2):707-723

[37] Chen D, McKearin D. Dpp signaling silences bam transcription directly to establish asymmetric divisions of germline stem cells. Current Biology. 2003;**13**(20):1786-1791

[38] Drummond-Barbosa D, Spradling AC. Stem cells and their progeny respond to nutritional changes during *Drosophila* oogenesis. Developmental Biology. 2001;**231**(1):265-278

[39] McLeod CJ, Wang L, Wong C, Jones DL. Stem cell dynamics in response to nutrient availability. Current Biology. 2010;**20**(23):2100-2105

[40] Bohni R, Riesgo-Escovar J, Oldham S, Brogiolo W, Stocker H, Andruss BF, et al. Autonomous control of cell and organ size by CHICO, a *Drosophila* homolog of vertebrate IRS1-4. Cell. 1999;**97**(7):865-875

[41] Britton JS, Lockwood WK, Li L, Cohen SM, Edgar BA. *Drosophila*'s insulin/PI3-kinase pathway coordinates cellular metabolism with nutritional conditions. Developmental Cell. 2002;**2**(2):239-249

[42] Cao C, Brown MR. Localization of an insulin-like peptide in brains of two flies. Cell and Tissue Research. 2001;**304**(2):317-321

[43] Brogiolo W, Stocker H, Ikeya T, Rintelen F, Fernandez R, Hafen E. An evolutionarily conserved function of the *Drosophila* insulin receptor and insulin-like peptides in growth control. Current Biology. 2001;**11**(4):213-221

[44] Ikeya T, Galic M, Belawat P, Nairz K, Hafen E. Nutrient-dependent expression of insulin-like peptides from neuroendocrine cells in the CNS contributes to growth regulation in *Drosophila*. Current Biology. 2002;**12**(15):1293-1300

[45] LaFever L, Drummond-Barbosa D. Direct control of germline stem cell division and cyst growth by neural insulin in *Drosophila*. Science. 2005;**309**(5737):1071-1073

[46] Rulifson EJ, Kim SK, Nusse R. Ablation of insulin-producing neurons in flies: Growth and diabetic phenotypes. Science. 2002;**296**(5570):1118-1120

[47] Smit AB, Vreugdenhil E, Ebberink RH, Geraerts WP, Klootwijk J, Joosse J. Growth-controlling molluscan neurons produce the precursor of an insulin-related peptide. Nature. 1988;**331**(6156):535-538

[48] Hetru C, Li KW, Bulet P, Lagueux M, Hoffmann JA. Isolation and structural characterization of an insulin-related molecule, a predominant neuropeptide from Locusta migratoria. European Journal of Biochemistry. 1991;**201**(2):495-499

[49] Kawakami A, Iwami M, Nagasawa H, Suzuki A, Ishizaki H. Structure and organization of four clustered genes that encode bombyxin, an insulin-related brain secretory peptide of the silkmoth *Bombyx mori*. Proceedings of the National Academy of Sciences U S A. 1989;**86**(18):6843-6847

[50] Masumura M, Satake S, Saegusa H, Mizoguchi A. Glucose stimulates the release of bombyxin, an insulin-related peptide of the silkworm *Bombyx mori*. General and Comparative Endocrinology. 2000;**118**(3):393-399

[51] Hsu HJ, LaFever L, Drummond-Barbosa D. Diet controls normal and tumorous germline stem cells via insulin-dependent and -independent mechanisms in *Drosophila*. Developmental Biology. 2008;**313**(2):700-712

[52] Ueishi S, Shimizu H, Y HI. Male germline stem cell division and spermatocyte growth require insulin signaling in *Drosophila*. Cell Structure and Function. 2009;**34**(1):61-69

[53] Amoyel M, Hillion KH, Margolis SR, Bach EA. Somatic stem cell differentiation is regulated by PI3K/Tor signaling in response to local cues. Development. 2016;**143**(21):3914-3925

[54] Cheng J, Turkel N, Hemati N, Fuller MT, Hunt AJ, Yamashita YM. Centrosome misorientation reduces stem cell division during ageing. Nature. 2008;**456**(7222):599-604

[55] Inaba M, Yuan H, Salzmann V, Fuller MT, Yamashita YM. E-cadherin is required for centrosome and spindle orientation in *Drosophila* male germline stem cells. PLoS One. 2010;**5**(8):e12473

[56] Yuan H, Chiang CY, Cheng J, Salzmann V, Yamashita YM. Regulation of cyclin A localization downstream of Par-1 function is critical for the centrosome orientation checkpoint in *Drosophila* male germline stem cells. Developmental Biology. 2012;**361**(1):57-67

[57] Roth TM, Chiang CY, Inaba M, Yuan H, Salzmann V, Roth CE, et al. Centrosome misorientation mediates slowing of the cell cycle under limited nutrient conditions in *Drosophila* male germline stem cells. Molecular Biology of the Cell. 2012;**23**(8):1524-1532

[58] Yamanaka N, Rewitz KF, O'Connor MB. Ecdysone control of developmental transitions: Lessons from *Drosophila* research. Annual Review of Entomology. 2013;**58**:497-516

[59] Baehrecke EH. Ecdysone signaling cascade and regulation of *Drosophila* metamorphosis. Archives of Insect Biochemistry and Physiology. 1996;**33**(3-4):231-244

[60] Carney GE, Bender M. The *Drosophila* ecdysone receptor (EcR) gene is required maternally for normal oogenesis. Genetics. 2000;**154**(3):1203-1211

[61] Mangelsdorf DJ, Thummel C, Beato M, Herrlich P, Schutz G, Umesono K, et al. The nuclear receptor superfamily: The second decade. Cell. 1995;**83**(6):835-839

[62] Hayward DC, Bastiani MJ, Trueman JW, Truman JW, Riddiford LM, Ball EE. The sequence of Locusta RXR, homologous to *Drosophila* Ultraspiracle, and its evolutionary implications. Development Genes and Evolution. 1999;**209**(9):564-571

[63] King-Jones K, Thummel CS. Nuclear receptors–a perspective from *Drosophila*. Nature Reviews Genetics. 2005;**6**(4):311-323

[64] Riddihough G, Pelham HR. An ecdysone response element in the *Drosophila* hsp27 promoter. EMBO Journal. 1987;**6**(12):3729-3734

[65] Cherbas L, Lee K, Cherbas P. Identification of ecdysone response elements by analysis of the *Drosophila* Eip28/29 gene. Genes & Development. 1991;**5**(1):120-131

[66] Dobens L, Rudolph K, Berger EM. Ecdysterone regulatory elements function as both transcriptional activators and repressors. Molecular and Cellular Biology. 1991;**11**(4):1846-1853

[67] Buszczak M, Freeman MR, Carlson JR, Bender M, Cooley L, Segraves WA. Ecdysone response genes govern egg chamber development during mid-oogenesis in *Drosophila*. Development. 1999;**126**(20):4581-4589

[68] Deng WM, Bownes M. Two signalling pathways specify localised expression of the Broad-Complex in *Drosophila* eggshell patterning and morphogenesis. Development. 1997;**124**(22):4639-4647

[69] Hagedorn HH, O'Connor JD, Fuchs MS, Sage B, Schlaeger DA, Bohm MK. The ovary as a source of alpha-ecdysone in an adult mosquito. Proceedings of the National Academy of Sciences U S A. 1975;**72**(8):3255-3259

[70] Handler AM. Ecdysteroid titers during pupal and adult development in *Drosophila melanogaster*. Developmental Biology. 1982;**93**(1):73-82

[71] Hodgetts RB, Sage B, O'Connor JD. Ecdysone titers during postembryonic development of *Drosophila melanogaster*. Developmental Biology. 1977;**60**(1):310-317

[72] Garen A, Kauvar L, Lepesant JA. Roles of ecdysone in *Drosophila* development. Proceedings of the National Academy of Sciences U S A. 1977;**74**(11):5099-5103

[73] Ables ET, Drummond-Barbosa D. The steroid hormone ecdysone functions with intrinsic chromatin remodeling factors to control female germline stem cells in *Drosophila*. Cell Stem Cell. 2010;**7**(5):581-592

[74] Xi R, Xie T. Stem cell self-renewal controlled by chromatin remodeling factors. Science. 2005;**310**(5753):1487-1489

[75] Konig A, Yatsenko AS, Weiss M, Shcherbata HR. Ecdysteroids affect *Drosophila* ovarian stem cell niche formation and early germline differentiation. EMBO Journal. 2011;**30**(8):1549-1562

[76] Morris LX, Spradling AC. Steroid signaling within *Drosophila* ovarian epithelial cells sex-specifically modulates early germ cell development and meiotic entry. PLoS One. 2012;**7**(10):e46109

[77] Li Y, Ma Q, Cherry CM, Matunis EL. Steroid signaling promotes stem cell maintenance in the *Drosophila* testis. Developmental Biology. 2014;**394**(1):129-141

[78] Yapici N, Kim YJ, Ribeiro C, Dickson BJ. A receptor that mediates the post-mating switch in *Drosophila* reproductive behaviour. Nature. 2008;**451**(7174):33-37

[79] Hasemeyer M, Yapici N, Heberlein U, Dickson BJ. Sensory neurons in the *Drosophila* genital tract regulate female reproductive behavior. Neuron. 2009;**61**(4):511-518

[80] Ameku T, Niwa R. Mating-induced increase in germline stem cells via the neuroendocrine system in female *Drosophila*. PLoS Genetetics. 2016;**12**(6):e1006123

Chapter 3

Primordial Germ Cell Reprogramming

Maria P. De Miguel, Yago Alcaina and
Diego Sainz de la Maza

Additional information is available at the end of the chapter

http://dx.doi.org/10.5772/intechopen.69965

Abstract

Primordial germ cells (PGCs) are the embryonic precursors of the gametes. Thus, they are unipotent cells. However, PGCs share some common features with pluripotent stem cells. Among them, PGCs show alkaline phosphatase activity and express stage-specific embryonic antigens and pluripotency factors Lin28, Oct4, Sox2, and Nanog. Under specific conditions, they undergo spontaneous reprogramming *in vivo*. Moreover, they can be easily reprogrammed *in vitro* into pluripotent embryonic germ cells (EGCs) by culturing them in the presence of basic fibroblast growth factor or the epigenetic modulator trichostatin A. Previous work in our laboratory has also proven that hypoxia alone can reprogram PGCs into hypoxia-induced embryonic germ-like cells, which have a pluripotent phenotype but which do not show self-renewal capacity. Therefore, PGCs are an interesting model to further comprehensively understand the process of cell reprogramming. This chapter reviews various methods to achieve PGC reprogramming, as well as the molecular pathways involved. We focus on soluble factors and genetic strategies to obtain pluripotent cells from PGCs. Special emphasis will be given to factors implied in energetic metabolism, epigenetics, and cell signaling transduction, both *in vitro* and *in vivo*.

Keywords: cellular reprogramming, ROS, glycolysis, autophagy, primordial germ cells, pluripotency, metabolism, hypoxia, epigenetics

1. Introduction

During normal embryogenesis and throughout the life of an organism, cells maintain or restrain their developmental potential. This potential refers to the ability to give rise to various types of cells. After fertilization, the resulting zygote and the blastomeres are totipotent until the four-cell stage, meaning they can develop a complete organism alone, including extraembryonic tissues such as the placenta [1]. Pluripotent stem cells, like embryonic stem cells (ESCs), are defined by their potential to differentiate into cells of the three germ layers (endoderm, mesoderm, and ectoderm), but they do not give rise to extraembryonic structures. In a more differentiated state, we find multipotent cells capable of differentiating into several types of cells. This capability is common in progenitor cells in adults, which give rise to diverse tissue cells.

In some processes, differentiated cells revert to a less differentiated and higher potential state. These phenomena are called reprogramming and are shown both *in vivo* and *in vitro*. *In vivo* reprogramming can be demonstrated by the appearance of cancer stem cells, and *in vitro* reprogramming has been achieved by several methods, such as somatic cell nuclear transfer, cell fusion between somatic and pluripotent cells, and treatment with pluripotent cell extracts, among others [2].

The most important and well-studied method of *in vitro* reprogramming in the last decade has been the derivation of induced pluripotent stem cells (iPSCs) from somatic cells by transduction of specific transcription factors, Oct4, Sox2, Klf4, and c-Myc [3]. These cells represented a revolution in stem cell research because they eliminated the ethical concerns about the use of ESCs and allowed access to an endless and personalized source of pluripotent cells. The clinical potential of this discovery is enormous, with the possibility of generating patient-derived iPSCs with applications not only in autologous transplants, but also in disease modeling and regenerative therapy. The use of iPSCs is extensive, and new ways to improve their derivation are being studied to increase efficiency and to overcome the risks for their clinical use. Even with the progress that has been made, there is still much to understand about the mechanisms of reprogramming.

In the study of pluripotency induction, an important model could be the use of primordial germ cells (PGCs), which can give rise to pluripotent cells called embryonic germ cells (EGCs). This reprogramming is achieved relatively easily, without the need for gene transduction, thus avoiding the risks related to gene manipulation [4–6]. PGCs are the embryonic precursors of gametes, giving rise during normal development to either spermatozoids or oocytes. These cells have limited self-renewal ability and are unipotent, are incapable of forming pluripotent embryoid bodies or contributing to teratomas or chimeras [7]. However, PGCs are considered developmentally pluripotent, given they generate the whole totipotent zygote after fertilization. This dual identity of both differentiated and pluripotent stem cells make PGCs a unique model to study cell fate and flexibility.

PGCs suffer reprogramming both *in vivo* and *in vitro*. *In vivo*, PGCs can give rise to embryonal carcinoma cells (ECCs), which are the pluripotent stem cells of testicular tumors [7]. *In vitro*, PGCs are easily reprogrammed into pluripotent EGCs with a specific cocktail of growth factors [4].

The reprogramming ability of PGCs can be explained by their similarity to pluripotent cells and their latent totipotency. PGCs innately express several transcription factors related to pluripotency, such as Oct4, Sox2, Nanog, and Lin28 [7]. Some of these factors are retained during PGC development from the zygote, whereas others such as Sox2, Nanog, and Klf2 are reexpressed or upregulated [8].

Other markers, such as tissue nonspecific alkaline phosphatase (TNAP) and germ cell nuclear antigen, do not belong to the pluripotency network itself, but are also strongly expressed by PGCs and ESCs. Even typical germ line factors such as B lymphocyte-induced maturation protein-1 (Blimp1) and Stella are typically expressed by ESCs [9]. It has been described that derivation of ESCs from the inner cell mass (ICM) is preferably achieved from cells that express Blimp1 and other germ line markers (interferon-induced transmembrane protein 3, Lin28, Prdm14, Stella, & c-Kit) [10]. The similarities in gene expression between PGCs and ESCs lead to the idea that the closest *in vivo* equivalent to ESCs are germ cells, instead of the ICM or even the epiblast, because PGC precursors are specified within the epiblast around 6 days post coitum (dpc) in mice [11].

The proximity of the PGCs to pluripotent stem cells and the ease of their reprogramming agree with the results of experiments on iPSC derivation from differently developed cells. The more undifferentiated the cells, the more easily they give rise to iPSCs, in a more efficient manner and requiring the transduction of fewer transcription factors. Conversely, the more differentiated cells, the more difficult they are to reprogram [12]. PGCs, however, can be reprogrammed with the transduction of only one of any of the four traditional iPSC factors [13]. This result is especially interesting because PGCs already express Oct4 and Sox2, which means that a variation in the expression level of just one transcription factor can be sufficient for PGCs to become pluripotent.

2. PGC reprogramming *in vivo*

ECCs are the stem cells of testicular tumors, which can be maintained indefinitely in culture as pluripotent cells. ECCs were first established as cell lines from mouse teratocarcinomas 50 years ago. In humans, the first teratocarcinoma cell lines isolated *in vitro* were TERA1 and TERA2, but their identity as ECCs was not discovered until some years later [14].

These pluripotent stem cells share most of their characteristics with ESCs, such as self-renewal capacity, specific markers, and the ability for differentiation to any cell of the organism [15]. The main difference from other pluripotent cells is that they are usually aneuploid. The malignancy of these cells is highly dependent on the microenvironment, as has been observed in chimera formation experiments: ECCs injected into mouse blastocysts can contribute to the development of a normal chimera, or in some cases to tumors. Another difference from ESCs is the very low efficiency in colonizing the germ line, which makes them less suitable for establishing mutant rodent lines [2]. Some authors define these cells as multipotent rather than pluripotent due to limitations in the differentiation potential, which is even more limited in human lines that often show no differentiation potential at all [14]. This potential has not been consistent, changing from one ECC line to another, and varying with culture conditions, such as the F9 EC line, which was considered nullipotent until the discovery of the induction of differentiation by retinoic acid (RA) exposure [16]. Considering the definition of pluripotency as the ability to differentiate into cells of the three germ layers, most ECC lines are pluripotent, but could be considered incompletely or partially pluripotent cells.

The germ line origin of the ECCs was proven using transgenic *Steel* (*Sl*) mutant mice. These mice, carrying a homozygous mutation in the *Sl* locus are unable to express stem cell factor (Kit ligand), a growth factor required for PGC survival and proliferation [17]. When embryonic gonads of the teratogenic mouse strain 129/Sv are transplanted to the adult testis, teratoma formation occurs in wild-type mice but not in *Sl* mutants, suggesting the Kit ligand is implicated in ECCs.

Most ECC lines are derived from early mouse PGCs (8.5–10.5 dpc), and spontaneous teratomas have been described to start around 12.5 dpc. PGCs lose their ability to reprogram *in vivo* after 12.5 dpc, which is coincident with the time the PGCs are able to give rise to EGCs *in vitro*. When 129/Sv 12.5 dpc gonads were transplanted into adult testes, teratomas appear at an 80% incidence, whereas when 13.5 dpc gonads were grafted, the tumor incidence decreased to 8%. The induction of these tumors is also related to the strain used, and is far less efficient in strains other than 129/Sv [14, 15].

In vivo reprogramming of PGCs to ECCs depends on a variety of genetic factors. The best known mutation that affects the development of mice teratomas is Teratoma (Ter) [18] in the RNA-modifying gene DND microRNA-mediated repression inhibitor 1 (Dnd1). In homozygous 129/Sv-Ter mice, teratoma incidence increases up to 75%. This reprogramming appears to be linked with proliferation, because the PGCs of these mice continue proliferating after 13.5 dpc, whereas unmutated PGCs enter mitotic arrest. The Ter mutation appears to be caused by the surrounding somatic cells instead of the PGCs themselves. In a similar manner, doublesex-related transcription factor 1 (Dmrt1) mutants also develop teratomas at a high rate in 129/SV mice, but unlike the Ter mutation, this effect is achieved by the loss of Dmrt1 in PGCs [19, 20].

Also related to PGC transformation is the phosphoinositide-3 kinase (PI3K)/protein kinase B (Akt) pathway, whose upregulation could lead to the appearance of ECCs. This outcome can be observed in the effect of the specific inactivation in PGCs of the tumor suppressor phosphatase and tensin homologue (PTEN), which leads to an activation of PI3K/Akt signaling, and, therefore, testicular teratoma formation [21]. Among the Akt targets is the tumor suppressor Trp53, whose deletion increases the incidence of testicular teratomas in mice [22].

Testicular cancers in humans are classified into three categories: (1) teratomas and yolk sac tumors that develop in fetuses and infants and are classified as nonseminomas, (2) adult testicular cancer, both seminomas and nonseminomas, which appear in men aged between 20 and 40 years, and (3) spermatocytic cancer, which affects elderly men [20]. The first two types have characteristics in common with mouse carcinomas. Teratomas and yolk sac tumors that arise early in human life are the most similar to the teratocarcinomas described in mice, even if normal karyotypes are present, and probably also originate from PGCs. With respect to adult human testicular tumors, the cellular origin of these tumors is carcinoma *in situ*, which is considered to develop early from the germ line due to the similarity to PGCs and gonocytes. Between these similarities, there is the expression of specific membrane markers, such as Kit or TNAP; stem and early germ cell genes, such as Nanog or Vasa; and genomic imprinting [23]. These cells can remain nonpathological until adult life and later develop into teratomas. Unlike the previous type, these cancer cells show chromosomal abnormalities, such as isochromosome of the short arm of the 12th chromosome (iso-12p) [24].

As in the mouse, the PI3K/Akt pathway is related to teratoma formation in humans. AKT1 overexpression, Trp53 deficiency and PTEN inactivation, or KRAS and NRAS mutations, which lead to activation of this pathway, correlate with testicular cancer formation. The Kit signaling pathway can also be implicated in the origin of human ECCs. Both KIT and Kit ligand (stem cell factor) mutations are related to human teratomas [19].

In addition, typical reprogramming factors such as Oct4 and Sox2 [3] are related to *in vivo* germ cell reprogramming. The Oct4 expression level appears to affect germ cell reprogramming *in vivo*, given its reported overexpression in both teratomas and adult testicular cancers [25]. On the other hand, Sox2 is only expressed in ECC, but not in PGCs or other testicular cancer cells [26].

The appearance of human testicular cancer has also been shown to be related to disturbances in the environment of the germ cells in the embryo, and in diseases such as cryptorchidism, gonadal dysgenesis, or estrogen exposure during pregnancy [27–29]. Estrogen upregulates c-Kit in the genital ridges, which leads to an increased proliferation of PGCs and reprogramming [30, 31].

3. PGC reprogramming *in vitro*

EGCs are derived *in vitro* from PGCs when cultured with a specific cocktail of growth factors: stem cell factor (SCF), leukemia inhibitory factor (LIF), and basic fibroblast growth factor (bFGF) [4, 5, 32]. EGCs are complete pluripotent cells, which are, like ESCs, able to give rise to all cell types in the organism and to fully contribute to blastocyst complementation, including contributions to the germline transmission [5, 32]. EGCs also share specific markers, such as stage-specific embryonic antigens (SSEAs), Oct4, Nanog, and TNAP, with other pluripotent stem cells [33].

EGCs were first derived from mice [4, 5] and then from various other animals [34]. EGCs have also been derived from human PGCs of around 5–10 weeks of gestation, providing a source of pluripotent stem cells and a good model of reprogramming [32].

Contrary to ECCs, EGCs are euploid and the primary difference between them and ESCs is the epigenetic state [7]. At the time of reprogramming, PGCs find themselves in different phases of the erasure and reestablishment of genomic imprints, and these epigenetic features are transmitted to the resulting EGCs. The epigenetic state of the PGCs is related both to the maintenance of the latent totipotency and to the inhibition of the stemness [35]. The manipulation of PGC epigenetics has proven the capability of reprogramming to EGCs (as we discuss later), showing how close these cells are to pluripotency.

Pluripotent stem cells can be found in various development states, with mouse ESCs representing the most undifferentiated, or naïve. This state is characterized by small, compact colonies; better survival when passaged as single cells; higher efficiency in chimera formation; shorter doubling time; and different culture condition requirements [36]. Human ESCs and mouse epiblast stem cells represent the most differentiated or primed state, characterized by larger flat colonies [37]. Human EGCs share some of their features with naïve stem cells, such as colony shape and culture requirements, and other features related to a more differentiated state, such as the lack of teratoma formation when injected into mice and low efficiency when derived from subculture [38]. This outcome shows how close PGCs are to totipotency and how useful they can be as a study model. The only major problem for this model is the availability of PGCs, which are scarce at the time when they are able to reprogram and are difficult to expand, because they only survive approximately a week in culture [33].

4. Classical PGC reprogramming mechanism

As we previously explained, PGCs can be cultured with LIF and SCF, maintaining their phenotype and promoting their survival for approximately a week [11]. When basic fibroblast growth factor (bFGF) is added to the media, reprogramming of the PGCs is induced. The mechanisms involved in this process are still not fully understood. Several signaling pathways and genes have been shown to be implicated, such as Blimp1 downregulation, PTEN inactivation, Klf4, and c-Myc upregulation, PI3K/Akt signaling activation, and transforming growth factor (TGF)β signaling, among others [21, 39–41]. Most of these mechanisms are also involved in iPSC derivation, indicating a common regulatory network between the various reprogramming processes [19].

The dynamics of the transition from a unipotent germ cell to a pluripotent stem cell have been studied [42]. Three phases have been described, which are similar to those in iPSC derivation [43], based on the loss of germ cell characteristics and the expression of pluripotency genes: induction, preparation, and maintenance. This change in gene expression is a gradual process that takes approximately a week to complete. In the induction phase, along with the upregulation of Klf4 and embryonic stem cell-expressed ras (Eras), some germ cell markers, such as Dnd1 and Ddx4, start to be downregulated. Surprisingly, a large amount of PGCs that begin the reprogramming die in this first step. Some pluripotent factors, such as Klf4 and Eras, begin to be upregulated in the early phase, but they do not reach their higher expression until later phases, when most pluripotent factors, such as c-Myc and Nanog, are upregulated. In the preparation phase, some pluripotent markers, such as Klf4, Nanog, and Zfp42, reach their highest expression level, whereas others, such as Klf9 and Sox11, continue their gradual upregulation. It is also interesting to notice the high expression in this phase of the Meis family of transcription factors, a family related to the maintenance of hematopoietic stem cells.

Compared with PGC reprogramming, the traditional iPSC derivation process is far longer, taking approximately 3 weeks to complete. One primary difference between the EGC and iPSC derivation processes is that in the latter, a mesenchymal-to-epithelial transition takes place in an early phase. The lack of that event in PGC reprogramming could be due to the lack of the inverse process (epithelial-to-mesenchymal transition) during PGC specification, which is contrary to most somatic cells [8]. Moreover, the activation of genes already expressed in PGCs, such as SSEAs or TNAP, takes place in this first phase. The preparation phase is characterized by the upregulation of Nanog (as in EGC derivation), Sall4, and Esrrb. Other genes reactivated after these are Rex1, Lin28, and finally, Stella, Dppa4, or Pecam, among others. Between the transduced factors, endogenous Oct4 is typical of the preparation phase, whereas endogenous Sox2 is necessary for the maintenance phase [8].

Inhibition of Blimp could be the primary mechanism of bFGF-mediated EGC derivation. Blimp is the key germ cell specification gene [44], which has a potent repressive function. Among its targets are c-Myc and Klf-4, two of the primary pluripotency transcription factors; thus, Blimp inhibition leads to their upregulation [39]. These factors are particularly important in the acquisition of pluripotency, and they are the factors not expressed naturally in PGCs. It has recently been reported that deletion of Blimp1 in PGCs is sufficient to cause the derivation of EGCs in culture without bFGF [45].

5. Non-classical PGC reprogramming

It has been shown that the PI3K/AKT signaling pathway is involved in PGC reprogramming *in vitro*. PI3K is activated not only by bFGF but also by LIF and SCF, the three factors needed for EGC derivation. One of its primary downstream effectors is Akt, also known as protein kinase B, which has been observed to improve EGC derivation efficiency when activated in PGCs, even allowing the reprogramming in late PGCs up to 14.5 dpc. [40]. The specific *in vivo* inactivation of the tumor suppressor PTEN in PGCs, which leads to PI3K/Akt signaling activation, and enhances both EGC derivation and testicular teratoma formation [21]. Among Akt targets is the tumor suppressor Trp53. Akt inhibits its transcriptional activity by preventing its phosphorylation and nuclear accumulation. Deletion of Trp53 increases the incidence of testicular teratomas in mice and is enough to cause PGC reprogramming in culture in the absence of bFGF [40]. Trp53 deletion has similar effects on iPSCs, enhancing their induction [46].

The cell proliferation rate also appears to be as important in PGC reprogramming as it is in iPSC derivation [47]. The time when PGCs have the highest potential to give rise to EGCs coincides with the moment of the highest proliferation *in vivo* [5]. The three growth factors typically used for EGC derivation are mitogens that can alone promote proliferation [48]. Also, bFGF can be replaced by other known mitogens, such as RA or forskolin [11, 49], which activates protein kinase A by increasing the intracellular cyclic AMP. These pro-mitogenic effects could be triggered both by MAPK signaling [50] and the PI3K/Akt pathway, which enhances proliferation through several downstream effectors. One is by the already mentioned inhibition of Trp53, but there are others, such as the activation of cyclin D and inhibition of cyclin-dependent protein kinase inhibitors (CDKIs) [51]. The effects of CDKI inactivation have been observed in the mutation of the CDKI inhibitor of CDK4 (INK4), which enhances teratoma formation in mice, along with Trp53 inhibition [22].

PGC reprogramming can also be achieved by inhibition of MAPK/extracellular signal-regulated kinase (ERK), and glycogen synthase kinase-3 (GSK3) signaling. The two inhibitors that have been used for this purpose have been PD0325901 (PD) and CHIR99021, respectively (named 2i), which in combination with LIF can replace both SCF and bFGF and give rise to EGCs [52]. The same inhibitors have been used to enhance iPSC derivation, thus obtaining a more undifferentiated phenotype [53]. The mechanism followed by 2i or by bFGF reprogramming differs, because bFGF activates MAPK signaling [54]. It has been proposed that MAPK/ERK inhibition can lead to pluripotency by promoting long-term self-renewal and inhibiting differentiation through downregulation of Lef1. In ESCs, Lef1 promotes differentiation by inducing lineage specific genes and suppressing pluripotency gene expression. On the other hand, GSK3 inhibits the Wnt/β-catenin pathway, being responsible for the Tcf3-mediated repression of other pluripotency-related genes, such as Sox2, Oct4, Nanog, and Esrrb [55, 56]. The difference between the mechanism triggered by bFGF and 2i is also revealed by the timing of the required compounds, whereas bFGF is only needed during the first 24 h [57, 58], continuous culture with 2i is required [52].

Recently, another glycogen synthase kinase 3 (GSK3) inhibitor has been found to achieve EGC derivation [41]: kenpaullone, which inhibits not only GSK3, but a wide spectrum of kinases such as CDKIs, and is sufficient for late (13.5–14.5 dpc) PGC reprogramming. Also, TGFβR inhibition by SB431542 can promote reprogramming in 11.5 dpc PGCs. The fact that these treatments have no effect on early PGCs, contrary to bFGF and 2i treatments, underlines the differences between the mechanisms that can trigger PGC reprogramming. TGFβ inhibition could induce reprogramming through promotion of proliferation [59], reducing MAPK activity [60], and directing induction of the pluripotency network. TGFβ inhibition can replace Sox2 transduction in iPSC generation by inducing Nanog expression [61]. On the other hand, the effect of various treatments can be combined to enhance reprogramming efficiency, such as TGFβR inhibition with 2i, with an efficiency of 12% [42]; TGF-β inhibition + ERK inhibitor (PD) [62], or bFGF + 2i + RA + forskolin, with an efficiency of approximately 20% [48]. This outcome shows that various mechanisms can synergize their effects in the reprogramming of PGCs. It has also been reported that mutations in genes involved in PGC development, such as Dnd1, Pten, and Pgct1, improve EGC derivation efficiency [19].

6. PGCs and hypoxia reprogramming

Recently, we have shown the reprogramming of PGCs cultured in hypoxic conditions without bFGF. The EGCs obtained had proven to be pluripotent, even if they were not completely reprogrammed, as shown by their limited proliferation [6].

The positive effects of hypoxia in enhancing reprogramming have been reported in iPSCs [63]. These hypoxia effects could be related to the idea of cancer stem cells arising *in vivo* from differentiated cells [64], due to environmental causes.

Hypoxia induces a change in the cell's energetic metabolism, from oxidative phosphorylation to glycolysis. This switch in the metabolism has been shown to be required for reprogramming of somatic cells to iPSCs. It has also been observed that the closest the somatic cell metabolism is to an ESC, the more efficient the reprogramming [65]. This metabolic change is an active process at the beginning of the reprogramming process; it has been shown that the expression of glycolytic genes, such as glucose transporter (Glut)1, Hxk2, Pfkm, and lactate dehydrogenase A (Ldha), is previous to pluripotency genes [66]. The relationship between stemness and glycolytic metabolism has been widely described in the Warburg effect, in which cancer cells in normoxia change their metabolism from oxidative phosphorylation to glycolysis [67]. It is still not clear whether the stem cell program triggers the metabolic change or whether it is the metabolic shift that activates the stem cell program; however, it has been demonstrated that these two processes are correlated. Our PGC data clearly supports the second hypothesis [6];

one described mechanism of this hypothesis is the positive feedback between glycolysis and the oncogene NF-κB [68].

The induction of PGC pluripotency by hypoxia has been demonstrated to be mediated by hypoxia-inducible factors (HIFs), given the inhibition of their degradation by dimethyloxaloylglycine mimics the effect of hypoxia in the EGC derivation. This agrees with the improved reprogramming efficiency observed in iPSC derivation when a prolonged expression of HIF1 is forced [69].

HIFs are transcription factors that regulate a large number of downstream effectors under hypoxic conditions. Among genes regulated by HIFs are pluripotency genes such as Oct4 and c-Myc, regulated by HIF2 or Notch, and ETS-1, regulated by HIF1 [70]. The metabolic switch can also be provoked by HIF activation. HIF regulates several metabolism-related genes, promoting the expression of glycolytic proteins such as GLUT1 & 3, LDHA, ENO1, aldolase A, phosphoglycerate kinase 1 (PGK1), glyceraldehyde 3-phosphate dehydrogenase (GAPDH), hexokinase 1 & 2, phosphofructokinase-2 (PFK2), and phosphofructokinase, liver type (PFKL)[65, 71].

These effects in the metabolism coincide with those provoked by Akt signaling, which is consistent with the mechanisms proposed for bFGF-mediated reprogramming of PGCs. Akt promotes glycolysis by the inhibition of FoxO transcription factors [51]. In somatic cell reprogramming, FoxO1 Akt-dependent phosphorylation enhances both glycolysis and iPSC derivation [72].

The mechanism by which HIFs provoke dedifferentiation in PGCs is partially known. It has been shown that the deregulation of Oct4 mediated by HIFs could be directly responsible for hypoxia-induced reprogramming [6]. Oct4 is one of the primary components of the pluripotency network; small changes in its expression levels result in great effects on stem cell development, promoting both undifferentiated and differentiated states, depending on the context [73]. Thus, in addition to the effect of its transduction on iPSC derivation, high levels of Oct4 can lead to differentiation and low levels can lead to pluripotency entry, provoking a dose-dependent induction of differentiation between mesoderm and trophectoderm in ESCs.

However, pluripotent hypoxia-derived EGCs cannot be passaged long-term, probably due to a lack of upregulation of c-Myc and Klf4. Gene expression analysis of these cells suggests that they have not reached the stabilization phase of cell reprogramming. Comparing the gene expression of these phases with those of hypoxia-derived EGCs has shown that the genes typical from initiation and maturation are upregulated; however, those belonging to the stabilization phase, such as Dppa3, Dppa4, Utf1, Eras, Lin28, Sox2, and Dnmt3l, are not [6].

As in 2i-mediated derivation of EGCs, and unlike bFGF, hypoxia is needed continuously to provoke PGC reprogramming. This need suggests a mechanism closer to that triggered by 2i. The relationship between hypoxia and GSK3 inhibition has been demonstrated by the fact that HIF1α stabilization depends on an inactive GSK3β pathway [74]. Under long hypoxia exposure, HIF1 is downregulated though activation of GSK3β. It has also been reported that Akt, which inhibits GSK3β, can upregulate HIFs through mammalian target of rapamycin (mTOR) activation [51]. This correlation supports the hypothesis of these two methods of PGC reprogramming, hypoxia and 2i, being connected.

7. Primordial germ cell reprogramming and energetic metabolism

Energetic metabolism has deep implications in germ cell development. As evidence, human PGCs show lipid droplets and glycogen accumulations on their cytoplasm in order to obtain energy [75].

Gene expression analysis comparing PGCs and EGCs showed no relevant differences in expression of pluripotency factors, whereas glycolytic enzymes displayed elevated levels in EGCs. This link between metabolism and PGC reprogramming has also been reported in PGCs cultured in hypoxia. This process leads to the induction of pluripotency, which is dependent on HIF1α stabilization and in turn provokes metabolic reprogramming and Oct4 deregulation [6]. Other studies have also observed that low Oct4 expression favors a robust pluripotent state in embryonic stem cells or acquisition of pluripotency, whereas high Oct4 levels relate to differentiation processes [76, 77]. In addition, Oct4, which remains active in PGCs, participates in metabolism regulation. In embryonic stem cells, Oct4 can induce hexokinase, pyruvate kinase, and pyruvate dehydrogenase (PDH) kinase expression, and the overexpression of these enzymes can prevent cell differentiation [78]. This has also been observed in PGCs [6]. In fact, when glycolysis is favored at low-oxygen concentrations, an increase in iPSC efficiency, and an enhancement of the expression of pluripotency factors via HIF expression are observed. Furthermore, iPSC derivation can be achieved in hypoxic conditions using only Oct4 and Klf4 [63, 79]. As mentioned for the comparison between PGCs and their *in vitro* pluripotent counterparts, EGCs, metabolism is also involved in the malignant transformation of PGCs into their pluripotent partners *in vivo*, ECCs. In particular, miRNA-regulated expression of enzymes involved in glycolytic metabolism contributes to the growth of germ cell tumors [80].

Oxygen levels are closely related to metabolism and potentiality. PGCs cultured in hypoxia are reprogrammed toward pluripotent cells and cause an increase in glycolytic genes, while they downregulate genes involved in oxidative phosphorylation (OXPHOS) [6]. Abundant evidence relates hypoxia to inhibition of oxidative metabolism. Among its effects, hypoxia inhibits cytochrome c oxidase and complex II of the electron transport chain. In fact, usage of the OXPHOS inhibitor carbonyl cyanide 3-chlorophenylhydrazone (CCCP) induces an upregulation of Oct4, Nanog, and Sox2 in embryonic stem cells [81]. On the other hand, culture of these cells in normoxia upregulates genes involved in differentiation [82, 83].

As previously mentioned, PGCs cultured in hypoxia give rise to pluripotent cells, and this process takes place in parallel with a metabolic shift toward glycolysis, which is governed by HIF1. Consequently, HIF1 inhibition disrupts PGC reprogramming, and HIF stabilization induces reprogramming [6]. HIF1 acts as a link between oxygen levels and metabolic phenotype inducing the expression of several genes related to glycolysis, such as glucose transporters, hexokinase, pyruvate dehydrogenase kinase 1, and lactate dehydrogenase. In fact, PGCs reprogrammed through culture in hypoxia show pyruvate dehydrogenase inhibition and mitochondrial inactivation [6]. Recent work from our laboratory has shown that PDH needs to be inhibited to achieve PGC reprogramming. Once the glycolytic profile is established under hypoxia, an increase in glycolytic flux through PKM2 activation renders in a synergetic effect with hypoxia (Sainz de la Maza et al. [129]).

Hypoxia can also alter the metabolic profile through mitochondrial mass modification. Mitochondria in pre-migratory PGCs are globular and localized around the nucleus. During migration, mitochondria increase in number and, when they undergo differentiation, they increase their number and size even further, and they acquire a more ovoid shape, further developing their cristae [84].

HIF1 inhibits PGC1β and induces mitophagy through Bnip3 upregulation [85]. In fact, autophagy is required in the early steps of cell reprogramming [86]. A shift has been reported in iPSC derivation from complex, active mitochondrial networks with developed cristae in fibroblasts to small, spherical, perinuclear, inactive mitochondria without cristae in pluripotent stem cells [66]. The results from our laboratory have shown that hypoxia-induced reprogramming causes a marked increase in Bnip3 expression, an essential gene involved in mitophagy. Autophagy takes places during reprogramming and is required for pluripotency acquisition (Sainz de la Maza et al. [129]).

Additionally, the Lin28/let7 pathway is crucial in glucose metabolism. In particular, Lin28 increases glucose uptake and metabolism through PI3K/mTOR activation and is involved in the translation of genes related to glycolysis, glucose metabolism, cellular carbohydrate metabolism, oxidative metabolism, and mitochondria in human embryonic stem cells [87–89].

Lin28 is also closely related to pluripotency, since it contributes to cell reprogramming and is present in the reprogramming cocktail, giving rise to iPSCs [90], and is also capable of activating the translation of Oct4 at the post-transcriptional level in human embryonic stem cells [91].

Primordial germ cells express Lin28 from 7.5 dpc in mouse PGCs and play a key role in Blimp1 expression. Lin28 is an RNA-binding protein that is able to bind the let7 precursor, impairing let7 processing. Therefore, miRNA let7 is not synthesized and is not able to inhibit Blimp1 translation; Lin28 indirectly stabilizes Blimp1 so PGCs can fulfill their germ cell specification [44, 92].

8. PGC reprogramming and epigenetics

PGCs undergo profound epigenetic reprogramming during their development [42]. Once specified, PGC express Blimp1, which is the master regulator of PGCs responsible for somatic program repression and germ cell identity [44]. In order to maintain Blimp1 expression and establish germ cell fate, Lin28 acts a negative regulator of let7 [92]. In human PGCs, Blimp1 is the effector that represses the somatic program, and Sox17 is the determinant transcription factor that establishes the germinal fate [93]. A recent study has shown a stable and elevated expression of Sox15 in early PGCs, which infers a possible role for this molecule in human PGCs as a master regulator, rather than Sox17 [94].

At the onset of specification, PGCs show several epigenetic marks, such as H3K4me2, H3K4me3, H3K9ac, H3K9me1, H3K9me2, H3K9me3, H3K27me2, and H3K27me3. However, these marks are shared at this time by neighboring, future somatic cells [95]. Once PGC migration begins, PGCs reduce the repressive mark H3K9me2 due to downregulation of the enzymes Ehmt1 and Ehmt2. PGCs also reduce DNA methylation by downregulation of the DNA methyltransferases Dnmt1, Dnmt3a, and Dnmt3b [8, 96]. Prdm14, an essential partner of Blimp1 in mouse germ cell development, and Tcfap2c intervene in this demethylation process downregulating Ehmt1, Ehmt2, Dnmt3a, and Dnmt3b. This partnership is also involved in the reexpression of transcription factors related to pluripotency, such as Sox2 and Klf2. However, Prdm14 is not necessary for human PGC development [97, 98]. PGCs progressively increase the repressive mark H3K27me3 via polycomb repressive complex 2 (PRC2) [95].

Later, once PGCs have reached the future gonads, they remove imprinting tags, increase H4R3me2 mark, and reactivate the inactive X chromosome in female PGCs [95, 99]. H4R3me2 modification, which takes place on arginine residues, is catalyzed by Prmt5, an epigenetic modulator that binds Blimp1, and exerts its epigenetic modifications until it is translocated back to the cytoplasm after E11.5 [100]. Another important event that occurs at this stage is major global DNA demethylation. It has been proposed that the vast extent of this DNA modification infers an active process and expression of the hydroxylase Tet1, the cytidine deaminase AID, and genes involved in base excision repair response (BER) have been detected. Nucleotide excision repair (NER) does not appear to be involved in PGC demethylation because no upregulation in molecules that take part in NER has been detected [101]. Finally, PGCs lose histone H1, increase nuclear size, lose chromocenters, reduce the epigenetic marks H3K9me3, H3K9me2, H3K27me2, H3K27me3, H3K9ac, and H4R3me2, and also lose nucleosomal, noncanonical histone H2a.Z [102, 103]. Blimp1 also induces the expression of Jmjd3 [104], responsible for removing the repressive epigenetic marks H3K9me2 and H3K9me3. In B cells, Blimp1 can also interact with chromatin modifier enzymes such as Kdm1a, a histone lysine transferase that catalyzes removal of methyl groups from lysines 4 and 9 of histone 3 [105]. In contrast to Blimp1, which appears to be essential in the repression of the somatic program, its effector Prdm14 contributes to establishing potential pluripotency through Sox2 upregulation in mouse PGCs, given that Sox2 is absent in human PGCs [97, 106]. Kdm6a is the histone demethylase that catalyzes the removal of the mark H3K27me3 during this second wave of reprogramming. The disruption of this process leads to an aberrant epigenetic reprogramming and loss of pluripotency markers Nanog, Oct4, and SSEA1 [107].

Sex determination begins at approximately E12.5. At this moment, DNA methylation is very low both in male and female PGCs [108, 109]. However, settlement of the epigenetic signature through DNA methylation occurs differently in male and female germlines. In males, *de novo* DNA methylation starts at around E13.5 and is accomplished before birth. Once methylation has been completed, gonocytes undergo vast proliferation and then they enter meiosis at the onset of gametogenesis. A disruption of methylation in male germ cells renders infertility [110]. In females, *de novo* methylation starts after birth and is not fulfilled until approximately P21 [111]. Oocytes undergo cell cycle arrest in meiotic prophase I, and it is not until ovulation that they re-enter meiosis. This coincides with the inability of PGCs to become reprogrammed.

Few studies have been performed on human PGCs, and the majority has focused on later stages of epigenetic reprogramming. Among the data available, early gonadal PGCs in humans (6–8 weeks of gestation) show low H3K9me2 and high H3K27me3 epigenetic markers [112]. Studies on pigs have also reported that changes in H3K9me2 and H3K27me3 markers are previous to DNA methylation, as observed in mouse PGC development [113]. Human PGCs also display active H3K4me1 and H3K4me3 marks and a peak in H3K9ac from 10 to 13 weeks of gestation. DNA showed a hypomethylated status and a loss of imprinting marks from gestation week 10 onwards. It is noteworthy that Blimp1 is restricted to the nucleus from week 7 to week 12, whereas Prmt5 is located in the cytoplasm, showing that there is no Blimp1/Prmt5 association in human PGCs [112].

Demethylated human PGCs later recover a methylated status, from week 13 of gestation to birth [114]. In addition, human postnatal gonocytes show a different epigenetic pattern from E13.5 mouse PGCs. Low levels of H3K9me2 are shared with mouse PGCs, but H3K27me3 shows low levels in post-migratory PGCs [112]. Also in contrast to mouse PGCs, the H3K9me3 repressive mark is observed in human gonocytes, as well as increased levels of H3K9ac active marks [115, 116]. Mouse PGCs show the lowest methylation at E13.5, when less than 10% of cytosines located at CpG islands are methylated [109]. Analyses of global methylation status from early stages of development have led to the observation that the ICM maintains its methylation status and, consequently, to the hypothesis that the germline is responsible for most of the DNA demethylation that takes place during development [117]. Specifically, the pattern appears to be a global demethylation during PGC migration, in which specific methylation marks in CpG islands (CGIs) of PGC-specific genes, CGIs on the X chromosome and differentially methylated regions in imprinted genes are conserved. Secondly, a new demethylation wave occurs when PGCs reach the genital ridges, affecting the previously mentioned sequences with epigenetic memory. This process involves both active and passive demethylation pathways [109]. Specifically, mouse PGCs fall from a 78% of global methylation at the epiblast stage to 5% at E11.5 (**Figure 1**). In human PGCs, demethylation takes place during the first 12 weeks of development, falling to 7% of methylation [118].

EGCs and ESCs can be fused to B-cells in order to originate a tetraploid hybrid. Methylation analysis has shown that the generated hybrids from EGCs showed lower methylation levels than those generated from ESCs, probably showing some sort of epigenetic memory in which EGCs resemble the low methylation status of their precedent PGCs. These hybrids eliminate the imprints that were present in ESC cells, suggesting that epigenetic reprogramming in EGCs is dominant over ESCs [119]. As previously mentioned, PGCs eliminate their imprinting marks at approximately E11-5. EGCs obtained from E11-5 or later PGCs also show demethylated imprinting marks, which cause serious alterations in developing chimeras [120, 121]. However, EGCs originated from previous PGCs show a less profound imprinting erasure and a more hypomethylated status regulated by Prdm14 when EGCs are cultured in the presence of GSK3β and MEK (2i) inhibitors [122, 123]. In fact, EGCs eliminate imprinting marks in the genes Igf2, Igf2rr, Dlk1, and H19, among others, which are established shortly after PGC specification [124, 125]. EGCs and ESCs also share as a common feature the activation of both X chromosomes in female cells [126].

PGCs can be reprogrammed into EGCs when cultured in the presence of trichostatin A (TSA), an inhibitor of histone deacetylase, in substitution for bFGF, stem cell factor and LIF [39]. In the case of bFGF, this growth factor needs to be added in the first

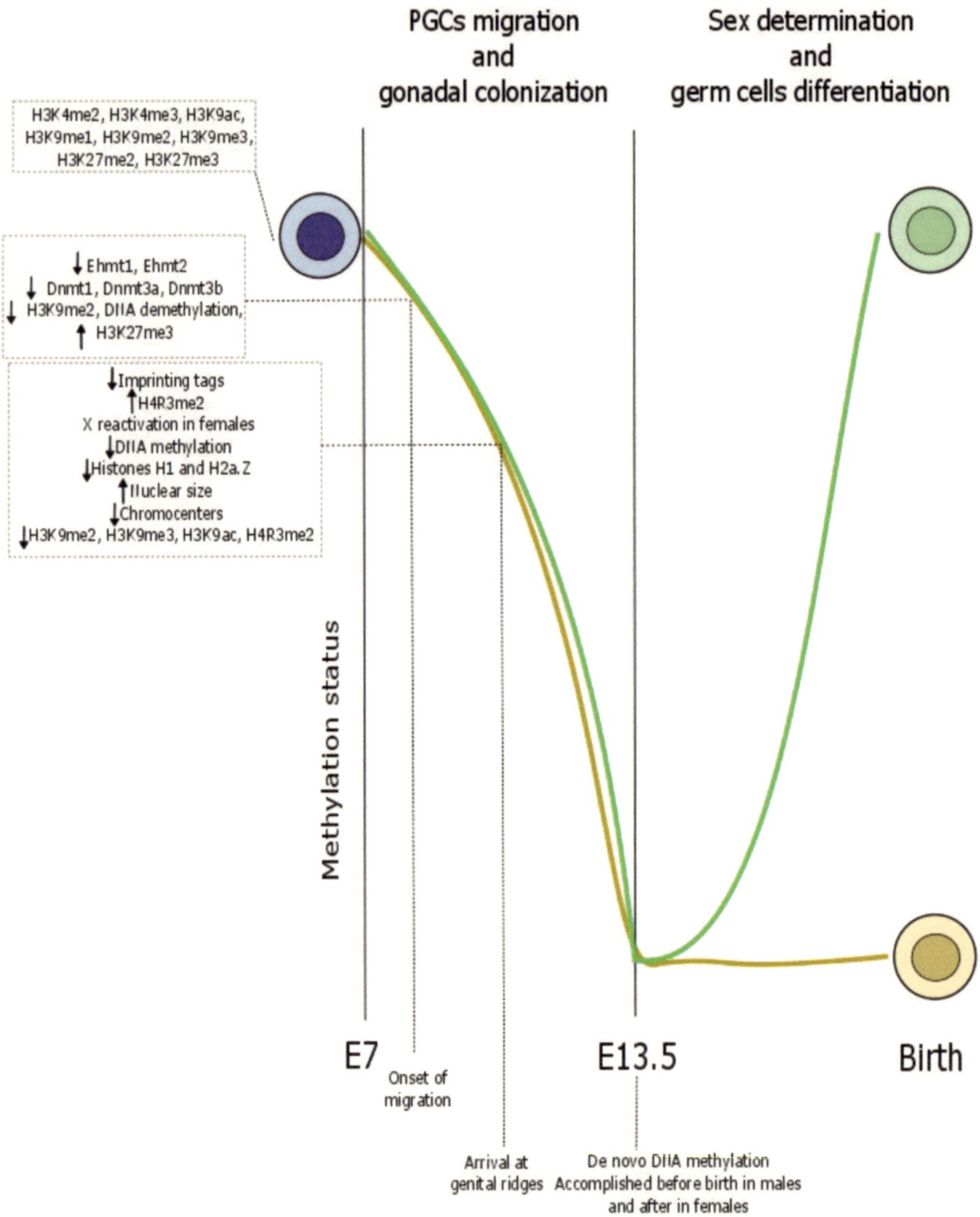

Figure 1. Modifications in DNA methylation during mouse PGC and gamete development. Both male and female germ cells share a first phase of epigenetic modifications, in which several processes lead to DNA demethylation and histone modifications. This phase corresponds to PGC migration and colonization of genital ridges in the first phase and development of gonads in the second. After sex determination, differential methylation is observed among male and female germ cells. Whereas male germ cells undergo *de novo* methylation at E13.5, female germ cells maintain hypomethylated status until birth.

24 h of culture. Substitution of bFGF by TSA accelerates the kinetics of EGC derivation, with a quicker downregulation of Blimp1 [39]. As stated in the classical PGC reprogramming section, bFGF-induced reprogramming of PGCs causes a downregulation of

Blimp1, which provokes an upregulation of Klf4, c-Myc, and Dhx38. This downregulation does not take place if bFGF is added later than 24 h of culture [39, 45, 127]. In EGC derivation by TSA, Blimp1 is absent in EGCs, whereas expression of Klf4, c-Myc, and Eras is detected. In bFGF-induced PGC reprogramming, Blimp1 disappears from PGC after 48 h [39].

As far as Prmt5 is concerned, this epigenetic modifier stays in the nucleus up to 7 days of culture, when it translocates from the nucleus to the cytoplasm in EGC colonies. Since Blimp1 binds Prmt5 to repress gene expression through H2A/H4R3me2s, contributing to maintaining the germ cell phenotype, absence of Blimp1 again appears to be a crucial event in PGC reprogramming. Direct targets of this mentioned repression, such as Dhx38 or c-Myc, are detected a few days after a bFGF-induced reprogramming procedure. These events were also observed in TSA-induced reprogramming of PGCs. [39]. Prmt5 has also been linked to pluripotency in ESCs. Its loss disrupts pluripotency and causes differentiation of these cells, where it is located in their cytoplasm [128]. Prdm14 is also essential for PGC derivation into EGCs. As previously mentioned, Prdm14 is an effector of Blimp1 and is involved in the downregulation of methylation enzymes during the first demethylation wave and in the reexpression of pluripotency factors. PGCs deficient in Prdm14 are unable to reprogram into EGCs because they cannot downregulate the repressive marker H3K9me2 and upregulate the epigenetic marker H3K27me3 via PRC2 [97]. Recent studies from our laboratory have shown that PRC2 is not involved in hypoxia-induced PGC reprogramming, whereas addition of histone deacetylase inhibitor valproic acid (VPA) is capable of inducing PGC reprogramming (Sainz de la Maza et al. [129]).

It is not surprising that epigenetic modifications relate to potency. Pluripotent stem cells show an open conformation of chromatin and active chromatin markers, such as H3K4me and H3K9ac [130, 131]. On the other hand, differentiated cells display repressed chromatin markers, such as H3K27me. Partially differentiated cells show a bivalent chromatin, with both active and repressing markers. Akt, one of the primary factors related to the reprogramming of PGCs, as noted before, also promotes a more active chromatin, mainly by inhibition of Mbd3, a component of the nucleosome remodeling deacetylase complex. Mbd3 is important in heterochromatin formation, and its inhibition promotes reprogramming in both EGC and iPSC derivation [19].

Epigenetics is also involved in the derivation of iPSCs. Fibroblast reprogramming can be achieved exclusively using soluble factors. In the reprogramming cocktail used by Hou et al [131], some epigenetic modifiers were included, such as the histone deacetylase inhibitors (HDACi) sodium butyrate and VPA, and the Kdm1a inhibitor tranylcypromine [132]. HDACi are strongly related to pluripotency acquisition. VPA has been proven to enhance iPSC generation, and usage of HDACi can turn pluripotent colonies with fuzzy edges into typical, compact pluripotent colonies [133–135]. VPA can also eliminate the imprinting marks located at the Dlk1-Dio3 gene cluster [136]. Inhibition of the polycomb complex, responsible for gene repression through DNA and histone methylation, results in lower iPSC derivation efficiency, probably because this complex is essential to the repression of the somatic program [137]. However, inhibition of histone methyltransferases by using BIX-01294 or inhibition of DNA methyltransferases using 5-azacytidine has been reported to improve iPSC derivation. The usage of BIX-01294 on fibroblasts with induced expression of only Oct4 and Klf4 rendered a comparable efficiency to that of using the four factors [138, 139]. A deeper understanding of the impact of epigenetics in reprogramming is required in order to elucidate the role of chromatin and histone modifications in the acquisition of pluripotency. Further research should be performed regarding the link between pluripotency and the germline program. For example, the induction of the expression of Prdm14, which is a Blimp1 effector, enhances iPSC derivation from mouse and human fibroblasts [140].

9. Concluding remarks and future directions

Various methods and soluble factors can be used for PGC reprogramming, including the classical bFGF [4, 5, 7, 141], the deletion of Trp53 [40], the addition of mitogens such as RA [11] or forskolin, [49], the inhibition of MAPK/ERK kinase and GSK3 signaling [52], and the addition of epigenetic modifiers such as TSA [39] and VPA (Sainz de la Maza et al. [129]). In addition, inducers of glycolysis such as hypoxia [6] and manipulation of cell metabolism are able to induce pluripotency (**Table 1**) and partial reprogramming, implicating many cytoplasmic and nuclear proteins (**Figure 2**).

All these data highlight the inherent potency of germ cells, allow for further and detailed characterization of the reprogramming process and are useful tools for the identification of genes involved in germ cell malignant transformation and the development of testicular tumors.

Method		Mechanism	Age (dpc)	Efficiency	Laboratory/year
bFGF		MAPK and PI3K/Akt activation	8.5	10/80	Hogan [5] and McLaren-Surani [58]
Forskolin		cAMP agonist	11.5	14.5 ± 3.9/(1/2 genital ridge)	Nakatsuji [49]
Retinoic acid		Mitogen	11.5	12.5 ± 5.2/(1/2 genital ridge)	Nakatsuji 1996 [49]
Trichostatin A		HDAC inhibitor	8.5	25/80	McLaren-Surani [58]
Valproic acid		HDAC inhibitor	8.5	ND	De Miguel, submitted
2i	PD0325901	MAPK/ERK inhibitor	8.5	9.4%	Smith [52]
	CHIR99021	GSK3β inhibitor			
SB431542		TGFβR inhibition	11.5	$2.08/10^4$	Nakano [41]
Kenpaullone		GSK3β and CDKs inhibitor	13.5	$2.27/10^4$	Nakano [41]
Hypoxia		HIFs activation	8.5	6.9%	De Miguel [6]

Table 1. Comparison of different methods of PGC to EGC reprogramming.

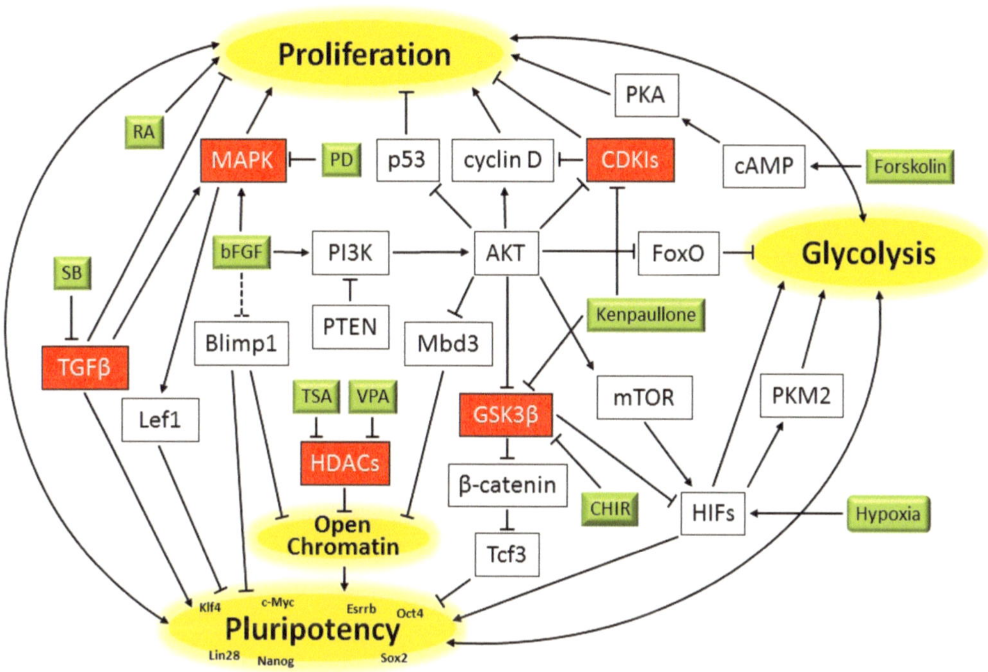

Figure 2. Schematic representation of the external factors (in green), signal transduction molecules (in red or white), and processes (in yellow) implicated in PGC reprogramming. Directly inhibited molecules in red. Arrows indicate induction and broken lines indicate repression of the pathway. PD: PD0325901; SB: SB431542; CHIR: CHIR99021; RA: retinoic acid; VPA: valproic acid; TSA: trichostatin A.

Acknowledgements

The authors thank financing from Roche Farma SA and Juliette Siegfried and her team at Servingmed.com for the English language editing.

Abbreviations

2i	two inhibitors (PD0325901 and CHIR99021)
BER	base excision repair response
bFGF	basic fibroblast growth factor
Blimp1	B lymphocyte-induced maturation protein-1
Bnip3	BCL2/adenovirus E1B 19 kDa protein-interacting protein 3
CCCP	cyanide 3-chlorophenylhydrazone
CDK4	cyclin-dependent kinase 4

CDKI	cyclin-dependent protein kinase inhibitor
CpG	cytosine phosphate guanine
Ddx4	DEAD-Box Helicase 4
Dlk1	delta like non-canonical notch ligand 1
Dmrt1	doublesex-related transcription factor 1
Dnd1	DND microRNA-mediated repression inhibitor 1
Dnmt	DNA methyltransferase
dpc	days post coitum
Dppa	developmental pluripotency associated
ECC	embryonal carcinoma cells
EGC	embryonic germ cells
Ehmt	euchromatin histone methyltransferase
ENO1	enolase 1Erasembryonic stem cell-expressed Ras
ESC	embryonic stem cells
Esrrb	estrogen-related receptor beta
FoxO	forkhead box class O
GAPDH	glyceraldehyde 3-phosphate dehydrogenase
Glut	glucose transporter
Hand1	heart and neural crest derivatives expressed 1
HDAC	histone deacetylase
HIF	hypoxia-inducible factor
Hxk2	hexokinase 2
ICM	inner cell mass of the blastocyst
iPSC	induced pluripotent stem cell
Jmjd	Jumonji domain containing
Kdm	lysine demethylase
Ldha	lactate dehydrogenase A
Lef1	lymphoid enhancer binding factor 1
Mbd3	methyl-CpG binding domain protein 3
MEF	mouse embryo fibroblast
Meis	myeloid ecotropic viral integration site
mTOR	mammalian target of rapamycin
NER	nucleotide excision repair
Oct	octamer-binding transcription factor
PARP	poly(ADP-ribose) polymerase
PDH	pyruvate dehydrogenase
Pecam	platelet endothelial cell adhesion molecule

PFK	phosphofructokinase
PGC	primordial germ cell
PGK1	phosphoglycerate Kinase 1
PKM	pyruvate kinase muscle
PRC2	polycomb repressive complex 2
Prmt	protein arginine methyltransferases
RA	retinoic acid
SCF	stem cell factor
SSEA	stage-specific embryonic antigen
Tbx3	T-box protein 3
Ter	teratoma
TGFβ	transforming growth factor β
TNAP	tissue non-specific alkaline phosphatase
TSA	trichostatin A
Utf	undifferentiated embryonic cell transcription factor
VPA	valproic acid
Zfp42	zinc finger protein

Author details

Maria P. De Miguel*, Yago Alcaina and Diego Sainz de la Maza

*Address all correspondence to: mariapdemiguel@gmail.com

Cell Engineering Laboratory, La Paz University Hospital BioMedical Research Institute, IDiPAZ, Madrid, Spain

References

[1] Nicholas JS, Hall BV. Experiments on developing rats. II. The development of isolated blastomeres and fused eggs. Journal of Experimental Zoology. 1942;**90**(3):441-459

[2] De Miguel MP, Fuentes-Julian S, Alcaina Y. Pluripotent stem cells: Origin, maintenance and induction. Stem Cell Reviews. 2010 Dec;**6**(4):633-649

[3] Takahashi K, Yamanaka S. Induction of pluripotent stem cells from mouse embryonic and adult fibroblast cultures by defined factors. Cell. 2006 Aug 25;**126**(4):663-676

[4] Resnick JL, Bixler LS, Cheng L, Donovan PJ. Long-term proliferation of mouse primordial germ cells in culture. Nature. 1992 Oct 08;**359**(6395):550-551

[5] Matsui Y, Zsebo K, Hogan BL. Derivation of pluripotential embryonic stem cells from murine primordial germ cells in culture. Cell. 1992 Sep 4;**70**(5):841-847

[6] Lopez-Iglesias P, Alcaina Y, Tapia N, Sabour D, Arauzo-Bravo MJ, Sainz de la Maza D, et al. Hypoxia induces pluripotency in primordial germ cells by HIF1alpha stabilization and Oct4 deregulation. Antioxidants & Redox Signaling. 2015 Jan 20;**22**(3):205-223

[7] Donovan PJ, de Miguel MP. Turning germ cells into stem cells. Current Opinion in Genetics & Development. 2003 Oct;**13**(5):463-471

[8] Kurimoto K, Yabuta Y, Ohinata Y, Shigeta M, Yamanaka K, Saitou M. Complex genome-wide transcription dynamics orchestrated by Blimp1 for the specification of the germ cell lineage in mice. Genes & Development. 2008 Jun 15;**22**(12):1617-1635

[9] Saitou M, Barton SC, Surani MA. A molecular programme for the specification of germ cell fate in mice. Nature. 2002;**418**(6895):293-300

[10] Chu L-F, Surani MA, Jaenisch R, Zwaka TP. Blimp1 expression predicts embryonic stem cell development in vitro. Current Biology. 2011;**21**(20):1759-1765

[11] De Felici M, Farini D, Dolci S. In or out stemness: Comparing growth factor signalling in mouse embryonic stem cells and primordial germ cells. Current Stem Cell Research & Therapy. 2009;**4**(2):87-97

[12] Kim K, Doi A, Wen B, Ng K, Zhao R, Cahan P, et al. Epigenetic memory in induced pluripotent stem cells. Nature. 2010 Sep 16;**467**(7313):285-290

[13] Nagamatsu G, Kosaka T, Saito S, Honda H, Takubo K, Kinoshita T, et al. Induction of pluripotent stem cells from primordial germ cells by single reprogramming factors. Stem Cells. 2013 Mar;**31**(3):479-487

[14] Andrews PW. From teratocarcinomas to embryonic stem cells. Philosophical transactions of the Royal Society of London Series B, Biological Sciences. 2002 Apr 29;**357**(1420):405-417

[15] Stevens LC. The development of transplantable teratocarcinomas from intratesticular grafts of pre- and postimplantation mouse embryos. Developmental Biology. 1970 Mar;**21**(3):364-382

[16] Strickland S, Mahdavi V. The induction of differentiation in teratocarcinoma stem cells by retinoic acid. Cell. 1978 Oct;**15**(2):393-403

[17] Donovan PJ, De Miguel MP. The role of the C-Kit/Kit ligand axis in mammalian gametogenesis. In: Matzuk MM, CW Brown, TR Kumar, editors. Contemporary Endocrinology: Transgenics in Endocrinology. Totowa, NJ: Humana Press Inc.; 2001. pp. 147-163

[18] Noguchi T, Noguchi M. A recessive mutation (ter) causing germ cell deficiency and a high incidence of congenital testicular teratomas in 129/Sv-ter mice. Journal of the National Cancer Institute. 1985 Aug;**75**(2):385-392

[19] Sekita Y, Nakamura T, Kimura T. Reprogramming of germ cells into pluripotency. World Journal of Stem Cells. 2016 Aug 26;**8**(8):251-259

[20] Kimura T, Murayama K, Nakamura T, Watanabe S, Umehara H, Tomooka M, et al. Testicular teratomas: Back to pluripotent stem cells. Progress in Molecular and Subcellular Biology. 2005;**40**:133-150

[21] Kimura T, Suzuki A, Fujita Y, Yomogida K, Lomeli H, Asada N, et al. Conditional loss of PTEN leads to testicular teratoma and enhances embryonic germ cell production. Development. 2003 Apr;**130**(8):1691-1700

[22] Sotillo R, Dubus P, Martin J, de la Cueva E, Ortega S, Malumbres M, et al. Wide spectrum of tumors in knock-in mice carrying a Cdk4 protein insensitive to INK4 inhibitors. The EMBO Journal. 2001 Dec 03;**20**(23):6637-6647

[23] Almstrup K, Hoei-Hansen CE, Nielsen JE, Wirkner U, Ansorge W, Skakkebaek NE, et al. Genome-wide gene expression profiling of testicular carcinoma in situ progression into overt tumours. British Journal of Cancer. 2005 May 23;**92**(10):1934-1941

[24] von Eyben FE. Chromosomes, genes, and development of testicular germ cell tumors. Cancer Genetics and Cytogenetics. 2004 Jun;**151**(2):93-138

[25] Rajpert-De Meyts E, Hanstein R, Jorgensen N, Graem N, Vogt PH, Skakkebaek NE. Developmental expression of POU5F1 (OCT-3/4) in normal and dysgenetic human gonads. Human Reproduction. 2004 Jun;**19**(6):1338-1344

[26] de Jong J, Stoop H, Gillis AJ, van Gurp RJ, van de Geijn GJ, Boer M, et al. Differential expression of SOX17 and SOX2 in germ cells and stem cells has biological and clinical implications. The Journal of Pathology. 2008 May;**215**(1):21-30

[27] Looijenga LH, Oosterhuis JW. Pathogenesis of testicular germ cell tumours. Reviews of Reproduction. 1999 May;**4**(2):90-100

[28] Kristensen DM, Sonne SB, Ottesen AM, Perrett RM, Nielsen JE, Almstrup K, et al. Origin of pluripotent germ cell tumours: The role of microenvironment during embryonic development. Molecular and Cellular Endocrinology. 2008 Jun 25;**288**(1-2):111-118

[29] Nistal M, Gonzalez-Peramato P, Regadera J, Serrano A, Tarin V, De Miguel MP. Primary testicular lesions are associated with testicular germ cell tumors of adult men. The American Journal of Surgical Pathology. 2006 Oct;**30**(10):1260-1268

[30] Moe-Behrens GH, Klinger FG, Eskild W, Grotmol T, Haugen TB, De Felici M. Akt/PTEN signaling mediates estrogen-dependent proliferation of primordial germ cells in vitro. Molecular Endocrinology. 2003 Dec;**17**(12):2630-2638

[31] Nistal M, Gonzalez-Peramato P, De Miguel MP. Sertoli cell dedifferentiation in human cryptorchidism and gender reassignment shows similarities between fetal environmental and adult medical treatment estrogen and antiandrogen exposure. Reproductive Toxicology. 2013 Dec;**42**:172-179

[32] Shamblott MJ, Axelman J, Wang S, Bugg EM, Littlefield JW, Donovan PJ, et al. Derivation of pluripotent stem cells from cultured human primordial germ cells. Proceedings

of the National Academy of Sciences of the United States of America. 1998 Nov 10;**95**(23):13726-13731

[33] De Miguel MP, Donovan PJ. Isolation and culture of mouse germ cells. Methods in Molecular Biology. 2000;**137**:403-408

[34] Miguel MPD, Kerr CL, López-Iglesias P, Alcaina Y. Techniques and conditions for embryonic germ cell derivation and culture. In: Kallos PM, editor. Embryonic Stem Cells - Basic Biology to Bioengineering. InTech; 2011;**22**:425-448, Michael S. Kallos (ed). Intech publishing, Rijeka, ISBN: 978-953-307-278-4. DOI: 10.5772/24632

[35] Surani MA, Hayashi K, Hajkova P. Genetic and epigenetic regulators of pluripotency. Cell. 2007 Feb 23;**128**(4):747-762

[36] Nichols J, Smith A. Naive and primed pluripotent states. Cell Stem Cell. 2009 Jun 05;**4**(6):487-492

[37] Tesar PJ, Chenoweth JG, Brook FA, Davies TJ, Evans EP, Mack DL, et al. New cell lines from mouse epiblast share defining features with human embryonic stem cells. Nature. 2007;**448**(7150):196-199

[38] Shamblott MJ, Axelman J, Littlefield JW, Blumenthal PD, Huggins GR, Cui Y, et al. Human embryonic germ cell derivatives express a broad range of developmentally distinct markers and proliferate extensively in vitro. Proceedings of the National Academy of Sciences of the United States of America. 2001 Jan 02;**98**(1):113-118

[39] Durcova-Hills G, Tang F, Doody G, Tooze R, Surani MA. Reprogramming primordial germ cells into pluripotent stem cells. PloS One. 2008;**3**(10):e3531

[40] Kimura T, Tomooka M, Yamano N, Murayama K, Matoba S, Umehara H, et al. AKT signaling promotes derivation of embryonic germ cells from primordial germ cells. Development. 2008 Mar;**135**(5):869-879

[41] Kimura T, Kaga Y, Sekita Y, Fujikawa K, Nakatani T, Odamoto M, et al. Pluripotent stem cells derived from mouse primordial germ cells by small molecule compounds. Stem Cells. 2015 Jan;**33**(1):45-55

[42] Nagamatsu G, Kosaka T, Saito S, Takubo K, Akiyama H, Sudo T, et al. Tracing the conversion process from primordial germ cells to pluripotent stem cells in mice. Biology of Reproduction. 2012 Jun;**86**(6):182

[43] Samavarchi-Tehrani P, Golipour A, David L, Sung HK, Beyer TA, Datti A, et al. Functional genomics reveals a BMP-driven mesenchymal-to-epithelial transition in the initiation of somatic cell reprogramming. Cell Stem Cell. 2010 Jul 2;**7**(1):64-77

[44] Ohinata Y, Payer B, O'Carroll D, Ancelin K, Ono Y, Sano M, et al. Blimp1 is a critical determinant of the germ cell lineage in mice. Nature. 2005 Jul 14;**436**(7048):207-213

[45] Nagamatsu G, Saito S, Takubo K, Suda T. Integrative analysis of the acquisition of pluripotency in PGCs reveals the mutually exclusive roles of blimp-1 and AKT signaling. Stem Cell Reports. 2015 Jul 14;**5**(1):111-124

[46] Krizhanovsky V, Lowe SW. Stem cells: The promises and perils of p53. Nature. 2009 Aug 27;**460**(7259):1085-1086

[47] Hanna J, Saha K, Pando B, van Zon J, Lengner CJ, Creyghton MP, et al. Direct cell reprogramming is a stochastic process amenable to acceleration. Nature. 2009 Dec 03;**462**(7273):595-601

[48] Leitch HGN, Nichols J, Humphreys P, Mulas C, Martello G, Lee C, Jones K, Surani MA, Smith A. Rebuilding pluripotency from primordial germ cells. Stem Cell Reports. 2013;**1**(1):66-78

[49] Koshimizu U, Taga T, Watanabe M, Saito M, Shirayoshi Y, Kishimoto T, et al. Functional requirement of gp130-mediated signaling for growth and survival of mouse primordial germ cells in vitro and derivation of embryonic germ (EG) cells. Development. 1996;**122**(4):1235-1242

[50] De Miguel MP, Cheng L, Holland EC, Federspiel MJ, Donovan PJ. Dissection of the c-Kit signaling pathway in mouse primordial germ cells by retroviral-mediated gene transfer. Proceedings of the National Academy of Sciences of the United States of America. 2002;**99**(16):10458-10463

[51] Manning BD, Cantley LC. AKT/PKB signaling: Navigating downstream. Cell. 2007 Jun 29;**129**(7):1261-1274

[52] Leitch HG, Blair K, Mansfield W, Ayetey H, Humphreys P, Nichols J, et al. Embryonic germ cells from mice and rats exhibit properties consistent with a generic pluripotent ground state. Development. 2010;**137**(14):2279-2287

[53] Silva J, Barrandon O, Nichols J, Kawaguchi J, Theunissen TW, Smith A. Promotion of reprogramming to ground state pluripotency by signal inhibition. PLoS biology. 2008 Oct 21;**6**(10):e253

[54] Eiselleova L, Matulka K, Kriz V, Kunova M, Schmidtova Z, Neradil J, et al. A complex role for FGF-2 in self-renewal, survival, and adhesion of human embryonic stem cells. Stem Cells. 2009 Aug;**27**(8):1847-1857

[55] Hackett JA, Surani MA. Regulatory principles of pluripotency: From the ground state up. Cell Stem Cell. 2014 Oct 02;**15**(4):416-430

[56] Ye S, Zhang T, Tong C, Zhou X, He K, Ban Q, et al. Depletion of Tcf3 and Lef1 maintains mouse embryonic stem cell self-renewal. Biology Open. 2017 Apr 15;**6**(4):511-517

[57] Donovan PJ, De Miguel MP, Hirano MP, Parsons MS, Lincoln AJ. Germ cell biology–from generation to generation. The International Journal of Developmental Biology. 2001;**45**(3):523-531

[58] Durcova-Hills G, Adams IR, Barton SC, Surani MA, McLaren A. The role of exogenous fibroblast growth factor-2 on the reprogramming of primordial germ cells into pluripotent stem cells. Stem Cells. 2006;**24**(6):1441-1449

[59] Godin I, Wylie CC. TGF beta 1 inhibits proliferation and has a chemotropic effect on mouse primordial germ cells in culture. Development. 1991 Dec;**113**(4):1451-1457

[60] Tan F, Qian C, Tang K, Abd-Allah SM, Jing N. Inhibition of transforming growth factor beta (TGF-beta) signaling can substitute for Oct4 protein in reprogramming and maintain pluripotency. The Journal of Biological Chemistry. 2015 Feb 13;**290**(7):4500-4511

[61] Ichida JK, Blanchard J, Lam K, Son EY, Chung JE, Egli D, et al. A small-molecule inhibitor of tgf-Beta signaling replaces sox2 in reprogramming by inducing nanog. Cell Stem Cell. 2009 Nov 6;**5**(5):491-503

[62] Attari F, Sepehri H, Ansari H, Hassani SN, Esfandiari F, Asgari B, et al. Efficient induction of pluripotency in primordial germ cells by dual inhibition of TGF-beta and ERK signaling pathways. Stem Cells and Development. 2014 May 15;**23**(10):1050-1061

[63] Yoshida Y, Takahashi K, Okita K, Ichisaka T, Yamanaka S. Hypoxia enhances the generation of induced pluripotent stem cells. Cell Stem Cell. 2009 Sep 4;**5**(3):237-241

[64] Krivtsov AV, Twomey D, Feng Z, Stubbs MC, Wang Y, Faber J, et al. Transformation from committed progenitor to leukaemia stem cell initiated by MLL-AF9. Nature. 2006 Aug 17;**442**(7104):818-822

[65] De Miguel MP, Alcaina Y, de la Maza DS, Lopez-Iglesias P. Cell metabolism under microenvironmental low oxygen tension levels in stemness, proliferation and pluripotency. Current Molecular Medicine. 2015;**15**(4):343-359

[66] Folmes CD, Nelson TJ, Martinez-Fernandez A, Arrell DK, Lindor JZ, Dzeja PP, et al. Somatic oxidative bioenergetics transitions into pluripotency-dependent glycolysis to facilitate nuclear reprogramming. Cell Metabolism. 2011 Aug 3;**14**(2):264-271

[67] Kondoh H, Lleonart ME, Nakashima Y, Yokode M, Tanaka M, Bernard D, et al. A high glycolytic flux supports the proliferative potential of murine embryonic stem cells. Antioxidants & Redox Signaling. 2007;**9**(3):293-299

[68] Kawauchi K, Araki K, Tobiume K, Tanaka N. p53 regulates glucose metabolism through an IKK-NF-kappaB pathway and inhibits cell transformation. Nature Cell Biology. 2008 May;**10**(5):611-618

[69] Mathieu J, Zhang Z, Nelson A, Lamba DA, Reh TA, Ware C, et al. Hypoxia induces re-entry of committed cells into pluripotency. Stem Cells. 2013 Sep;**31**(9):1737-1748

[70] Simon MC, Keith B. The role of oxygen availability in embryonic development and stem cell function. Nature Reviews Molecular Cell Biology. 2008 Apr;**9**(4):285-296

[71] Shaw RJ. Glucose metabolism and cancer. Current Opinion in Cell Biology. 2006; **18**(6):598-608

[72] Yu Y, Liang D, Tian Q, Chen X, Jiang B, Chou BK, et al. Stimulation of somatic cell reprogramming by ERas-Akt-FoxO1 signaling axis. Stem Cells. 2014 Feb;**32**(2):349-363

[73] Sterneckert J, Hoing S, Scholer HR. Concise review: Oct4 and more: The reprogramming expressway. Stem Cells. 2012 Jan;**30**(1):15-21

[74] Mottet D, Dumont V, Deccache Y, Demazy C, Ninane N, Raes M, et al. Regulation of hypoxia-inducible factor-1alpha protein level during hypoxic conditions by the phosphatidylinositol 3-kinase/Akt/glycogen synthase kinase 3beta pathway in HepG2 cells. The Journal of Biological Chemistry. 2003;**278**(33):31277-31285

[75] Fujimoto T, Miyayama Y, Fuyuta M. The origin, migration and fine morphology of human primordial germ cells. The Anatomical Record. 1977 Jul;**188**(3):315-330

[76] Radzisheuskaya A, Chia Gle B, dos Santos RL, Theunissen TW, Castro LF, Nichols J, et al. A defined Oct4 level governs cell state transitions of pluripotency entry and differentiation into all embryonic lineages. Nature Cell Biology. 2013 Jun;**15**(6):579-590

[77] Karwacki-Neisius V, Goke J, Osorno R, Halbritter F, Ng JH, Weisse AY, et al. Reduced Oct4 expression directs a robust pluripotent state with distinct signaling activity and increased enhancer occupancy by Oct4 and Nanog. Cell Stem Cell. 2013 May 2;**12**(5):531-545

[78] Kim H, Jang H, Kim TW, Kang BH, Lee SE, Jeon YK, et al. Core pluripotency factors directly regulate metabolism in embryonic stem cell to maintain pluripotency. Stem Cells. 2015 Sep;**33**(9):2699-2711

[79] Forristal CE, Wright KL, Hanley NA, Oreffo RO, Houghton FD. Hypoxia inducible factors regulate pluripotency and proliferation in human embryonic stem cells cultured at reduced oxygen tensions. Reproduction. 2010 Jan;**139**(1):85-97

[80] Liu X, Duan H, Zhou S, Liu Z, Wu D, Zhao T, et al. microRNA-199a-3p functions as tumor suppressor by regulating glucose metabolism in testicular germ cell tumors. Molecular Medicine Reports. 2016 Sep;**14**(3):2311-2320

[81] Mandal S, Lindgren AG, Srivastava AS, Clark AT, Banerjee U. Mitochondrial function controls proliferation and early differentiation potential of embryonic stem cells. Stem Cells. 2011 Mar;**29**(3):486-495

[82] Westfall SD, Sachdev S, Das P, Hearne LB, Hannink M, Roberts RM, et al. Identification of oxygen-sensitive transcriptional programs in human embryonic stem cells. Stem Cells and Development. 2008 Oct;**17**(5):869-881

[83] Lengner CJ, Gimelbrant AA, Erwin JA, Cheng AW, Guenther MG, Welstead GG, et al. Derivation of pre-X inactivation human embryonic stem cells under physiological oxygen concentrations. Cell. 2010 May 28;**141**(5):872-883

[84] Motta PM, Nottola SA, Makabe S, Heyn R. Mitochondrial morphology in human fetal and adult female germ cells. Human Reproduction. 2000 Jul;**15**(Suppl 2):129-147

[85] Zhang H, Bosch-Marce M, Shimoda LA, Tan YS, Baek JH, Wesley JB, et al. Mitochondrial autophagy is an HIF-1-dependent adaptive metabolic response to hypoxia. The Journal of Biological Chemistry. 2008 Apr 18;**283**(16):10892-10903

[86] Wang S, Xia P, Ye B, Huang G, Liu J, Fan Z. Transient activation of autophagy via Sox2-mediated suppression of mTOR is an important early step in reprogramming to pluripotency. Cell Stem Cell. 2013 Nov 07;**13**(5):617-625

[87] Polesskaya A, Cuvellier S, Naguibneva I, Duquet A, Moss EG, Harel-Bellan A. Lin-28 binds IGF-2 mRNA and participates in skeletal myogenesis by increasing translation efficiency. Genes & Development. 2007 May 01;**21**(9):1125-1138

[88] Peng S, Chen LL, Lei XX, Yang L, Lin H, Carmichael GG, et al. Genome-wide studies reveal that Lin28 enhances the translation of genes important for growth and survival of human embryonic stem cells. Stem Cells. 2011 Mar;**29**(3):496-504

[89] Zhu H, Shyh-Chang N, Segre AV, Shinoda G, Shah SP, Einhorn WS, et al. The Lin28/let-7 axis regulates glucose metabolism. Cell. 2011 Sep 30;**147**(1):81-94

[90] Yu J, Vodyanik MA, Smuga-Otto K, Antosiewicz-Bourget J, Frane JL, Tian S, et al. Induced pluripotent stem cell lines derived from human somatic cells. Science. 2007 Dec 21;**318**(5858):1917-1920

[91] Qiu C, Ma Y, Wang J, Peng S, Huang Y. Lin28-mediated post-transcriptional regulation of Oct4 expression in human embryonic stem cells. Nucleic Acids Research. 2010 Mar;**38**(4):1240-1248

[92] West JA, Viswanathan SR, Yabuuchi A, Cunniff K, Takeuchi A, Park IH, et al. A role for Lin28 in primordial germ-cell development and germ-cell malignancy. Nature. 2009 Aug 13;**460**(7257):909-913

[93] Irie N, Weinberger L, Tang WW, Kobayashi T, Viukov S, Manor YS, et al. SOX17 is a critical specifier of human primordial germ cell fate. Cell. 2015 Jan 15;**160**(1-2):253-268

[94] Guo F, Yan L, Guo H, Li L, Hu B, Zhao Y, et al. The transcriptome and DNA methylome landscapes of human primordial germ cells. Cell. 2015 Jun 04;**161**(6):1437-1452

[95] Seki Y, Yamaji M, Yabuta Y, Sano M, Shigeta M, Matsui Y, et al. Cellular dynamics associated with the genome-wide epigenetic reprogramming in migrating primordial germ cells in mice. Development. 2007 Jul;**134**(14):2627-2638

[96] Yabuta Y, Kurimoto K, Ohinata Y, Seki Y, Saitou M. Gene expression dynamics during germline specification in mice identified by quantitative single-cell gene expression profiling. Biology of Reproduction. 2006 Nov;**75**(5):705-716

[97] Yamaji M, Seki Y, Kurimoto K, Yabuta Y, Yuasa M, Shigeta M, et al. Critical function of Prdm14 for the establishment of the germ cell lineage in mice. Nature Genetics. 2008 Aug;**40**(8):1016-1022

[98] Sugawa F, Arauzo-Bravo MJ, Yoon J, Kim KP, Aramaki S, Wu G, et al. Human primordial germ cell commitment in vitro associates with a unique PRDM14 expression profile. The EMBO Journal. 2015 Apr 15;**34**(8):1009-1024

[99] Sasaki H, Matsui Y. Epigenetic events in mammalian germ-cell development: Reprogramming and beyond. Nature Reviews Genetics. 2008 Feb;**9**(2):129-140

[100] Ancelin K, Lange UC, Hajkova P, Schneider R, Bannister AJ, Kouzarides T, et al. Blimp1 associates with Prmt5 and directs histone arginine methylation in mouse germ cells. Nature Cell Biology. 2006 Jun;**8**(6):623-630

[101] Hajkova P, Jeffries SJ, Lee C, Miller N, Jackson SP, Surani MA. Genome-wide reprogramming in the mouse germ line entails the base excision repair pathway. Science. 2010 Jul 02;**329**(5987):78-82

[102] De Felici M. Nuclear reprogramming in mouse primordial germ cells: Epigenetic contribution. Stem Cells International. 2011;**2011**:425863

[103] Hajkova P, Ancelin K, Waldmann T, Lacoste N, Lange UC, Cesari F, et al. Chromatin dynamics during epigenetic reprogramming in the mouse germ line. Nature. 2008 Apr 17;**452**(7189):877-881

[104] Gunesdogan U, Magnusdottir E, Surani MA. Primordial germ cell specification: A context-dependent cellular differentiation event [corrected]. Philosophical transactions of the Royal Society of London Series B, Biological sciences. 2014 Dec 5;**369**:1657-1665

[105] Su ST, Ying HY, Chiu YK, Lin FR, Chen MY, Lin KI. Involvement of histone demethylase LSD1 in Blimp-1-mediated gene repression during plasma cell differentiation. Molecular and Cellular Biology. 2009 Mar;**29**(6):1421-1431

[106] Perrett RM, Turnpenny L, Eckert JJ, O'Shea M, Sonne SB, Cameron IT, et al. The early human germ cell lineage does not express SOX2 during in vivo development or upon in vitro culture. Biology of Reproduction. 2008 May;**78**(5):852-858

[107] Mansour AA, Gafni O, Weinberger L, Zviran A, Ayyash M, Rais Y, et al. The H3K27 demethylase Utx regulates somatic and germ cell epigenetic reprogramming. Nature. 2012 Aug 16;**488**(7411):409-413

[108] Guibert S, Forne T, Weber M. Global profiling of DNA methylation erasure in mouse primordial germ cells. Genome Research. 2012 Apr;**22**(4):633-641

[109] Seisenberger S, Andrews S, Krueger F, Arand J, Walter J, Santos F, et al. The dynamics of genome-wide DNA methylation reprogramming in mouse primordial germ cells. Molecular Cell. 2012 Dec 28;**48**(6):849-862

[110] Stewart KR, Veselovska L, Kelsey G. Establishment and functions of DNA methylation in the germline. Epigenomics. 2016 Oct;**8**(10):1399-1413

[111] Smallwood SA, Tomizawa S, Krueger F, Ruf N, Carli N, Segonds-Pichon A, et al. Dynamic CpG island methylation landscape in oocytes and preimplantation embryos. Nature Genetics. 2011 Jun 26;**43**(8):811-814

[112] Eguizabal C, Herrera L, De Onate L, Montserrat N, Hajkova P, Izpisua Belmonte JC. Characterization of the epigenetic changes during human gonadal primordial germ cells reprogramming. Stem Cells. 2016 Sep;**34**(9):2418-2428

[113] Hyldig SM, Ostrup O, Vejlsted M, Thomsen PD. Changes of DNA methylation level and spatial arrangement of primordial germ cells in embryonic day 15 to embryonic day 28 pig embryos. Biology of Reproduction. 2011 Jun;**84**(6):1087-1093

[114] Wermann H, Stoop H, Gillis AJ, Honecker F, van Gurp RJ, Ammerpohl O, et al. Global DNA methylation in fetal human germ cells and germ cell tumours: Association with differentiation and cisplatin resistance. The Journal of Pathology. 2010 Aug;**221**(4):433-442

[115] Almstrup K, Nielsen JE, Mlynarska O, Jansen MT, Jorgensen A, Skakkebaek NE, et al. Carcinoma in situ testis displays permissive chromatin modifications similar to immature foetal germ cells. British Journal of Cancer. 2010 Oct 12;**103**(8):1269-1276

[116] Bartkova J, Moudry P, Hodny Z, Lukas J, Rajpert-De Meyts E, Bartek J. Heterochromatin marks HP1gamma, HP1alpha and H3K9me3, and DNA damage response activation in human testis development and germ cell tumours. International Journal of Andrology. 2011 Aug;**34**(4 Pt 2):e103-e113

[117] Gkountela S, Zhang KX, Shafiq TA, Liao WW, Hargan-Calvopina J, Chen PY, et al. DNA demethylation dynamics in the human prenatal germline. Cell. 2015 Jun 04;**161**(6): 1425-1436

[118] Guo H, Hu B, Yan L, Yong J, Wu Y, Gao Y, et al. DNA methylation and chromatin accessibility profiling of mouse and human fetal germ cells. Cell Research. 2017 Feb;**27** (2):165-183

[119] Tada M, Takahama Y, Abe K, Nakatsuji N, Tada T. Nuclear reprogramming of somatic cells by in vitro hybridization with ES cells. Current Biology. 2001 Oct 02;**11**(19): 1553-1558

[120] Labosky PA, Barlow DP, Hogan BL. Mouse embryonic germ (EG) cell lines: Transmission through the germline and differences in the methylation imprint of insulin-like growth factor 2 receptor (Igf2r) gene compared with embryonic stem (ES) cell lines. Development. 1994 Nov;**120**(11):3197-3204

[121] Tada T, Tada M, Hilton K, Barton SC, Sado T, Takagi N, et al. Epigenotype switching of imprintable loci in embryonic germ cells. Development Genes and Evolution. 1998 Feb;**207**(8):551-561

[122] Shovlin TC, Durcova-Hills G, Surani A, McLaren A. Heterogeneity in imprinted methylation patterns of pluripotent embryonic germ cells derived from pre-migratory mouse germ cells. Developmental Biology. 2008 Jan 15;**313**(2):674-681

[123] Leitch HG, Tang WW, Surani MA. Primordial germ-cell development and epigenetic reprogramming in mammals. Current Topics in Developmental Biology. 2013;**104**:149-187

[124] Durcova-Hills G, Ainscough J, McLaren A. Pluripotential stem cells derived from migrating primordial germ cells. Differentiation. 2001 Oct;**68**(4-5):220-226

[125] Lee J, Inoue K, Ono R, Ogonuki N, Kohda T, Kaneko-Ishino T, et al. Erasing genomic imprinting memory in mouse clone embryos produced from day 11.5 primordial germ cells. Development. 2002 Apr;**129**(8):1807-1817

[126] Sharova LV, Sharov AA, Piao Y, Shaik N, Sullivan T, Stewart CL, et al. Global gene expression profiling reveals similarities and differences among mouse pluripotent stem cells of different origins and strains. Developmental Biology. 2007 Jul 15;**307**(2): 446-459

[127] Saitou M, Yamaji M. Primordial germ cells in mice. Cold Spring Harbor perspectives in biology. 2012 Nov 01;**4**(11):1-19

[128] Surani MA, Durcova-Hills G, Hajkova P, Hayashi K, Tee WW. Germ line, stem cells, and epigenetic reprogramming. Cold Spring Harbor Symposia on Quantitative Biology. 2008;**73**:9-15

[129] Sainz de la Maza et al. Metabolic reprogramming, autophagy, and reactive oxygen species are necessary for primordial germ cell reprogramming into pluripotency. Oxidative Medicine and Cellular Longevity. 2017;**2017**:Article ID 4745252. p. 17. DOI:10.1155/2017/4745252

[130] Meissner A. Epigenetic modifications in pluripotent and differentiated cells. Nature Biotechnology. 2010 Oct;**28**(10):1079-1088

[131] Gaspar-Maia A, Alajem A, Meshorer E, Ramalho-Santos M. Open chromatin in pluripotency and reprogramming. Nature Reviews Molecular Cell Biology. 2011 Jan;**12**(1):36-47

[132] Hou P, Li Y, Zhang X, Liu C, Guan J, Li H, et al. Pluripotent stem cells induced from mouse somatic cells by small-molecule compounds. Science. 2013 Aug 9;**341**(6146):651-654

[133] Huangfu D, Maehr R, Guo W, Eijkelenboom A, Snitow M, Chen AE, et al. Induction of pluripotent stem cells by defined factors is greatly improved by small-molecule compounds. Nature Biotechnology. 2008 Jul;**26**(7):795-797

[134] Tonge PD, Corso AJ, Monetti C, Hussein SM, Puri MC, Michael IP, et al. Divergent reprogramming routes lead to alternative stem-cell states. Nature. 2014 Dec 11;**516**(7530):192-197

[135] Chen X, Zhai Y, Yu D, Cui J, Hu JF, Li W. Valproic acid enhances iPSC induction from human bone marrow-derived cells through the suppression of reprogramming-induced senescence. Journal of Cellular Physiology. 2016 Aug;**231**(8):1719-1727

[136] Stadtfeld M, Apostolou E, Akutsu H, Fukuda A, Follett P, Natesan S, et al. Aberrant silencing of imprinted genes on chromosome 12qF1 in mouse induced pluripotent stem cells. Nature. 2010 May 13;**465**(7295):175-181

[137] Onder TT, Kara N, Cherry A, Sinha AU, Zhu N, Bernt KM, et al. Chromatin-modifying enzymes as modulators of reprogramming. Nature. 2012 Mar 04;**483**(7391):598-602

[138] Mikkelsen TS, Hanna J, Zhang X, Ku M, Wernig M, Schorderet P, et al. Dissecting direct reprogramming through integrative genomic analysis. Nature. 2008 Jul 03;**454**(7200): 49-55

[139] Shi Y, Desponts C, Do JT, Hahm HS, Scholer HR, Ding S. Induction of pluripotent stem cells from mouse embryonic fibroblasts by Oct4 and Klf4 with small-molecule compounds. Cell Stem Cell. 2008 Nov 6;**3**(5):568-574

[140] Chia NY, Chan YS, Feng B, Lu X, Orlov YL, Moreau D, et al. A genome-wide RNAi screen reveals determinants of human embryonic stem cell identity. Nature. 2010 Nov 11;**468**(7321):316-320

[141] Donovan PJ, Stott D, Cairns LA, Heasman J, Wylie CC. Migratory and postmigratory mouse primordial germ cells behave differently in culture. Cell. 1986;**44**(6):831-838

Chapter 4

Membrane Dynamics of Spermatozoa during Capacitation: New Insight in Germ Cells Signalling

Nicola Bernabò, Marina Ramal Sanchez,
Luca Valbonetti, Luana Greco, Giulia Capacchietti,
Mauro Mattioli and Barbara Barboni

Additional information is available at the end of the chapter

http://dx.doi.org/10.5772/intechopen.69964

Abstract

The study of germline stem cells and of germline cells has deep implications for the understanding of fertility, development and cancer. Nowadays, we are experiencing the very fascinating challenge of application of *–OMICS* technologies to this issue, which is opening new and unexpected horizons in virtually all the branches of biology. Here, we carried out a review of signalling systems involved in maturation of male germ cells and in the process that leads them to become fully fertile. In particular, we discuss the control mechanisms involved in capacitation and acrosome reaction that act at membrane level. Indeed, spermatozoa membranes play key roles in determining the achievement of fertility: they are the interface with the surrounding environment, they locate the signal transduction systems and they are active in recognizing and binding the oocyte. In addition, we discuss the effect of several compounds that could exert a negative effect on reproductive activity, by interfering with the endocrine axis, the so-called endocrine disruptors.

Keywords: germline stem cells, spermatozoa, membrane, signalling, fertility

1. Introduction

In recent years, the scientific interest for germline stem cells (GSCs) has enormously grown. They are the cells devoted to the genome transmission to future generations; thus the study of their biology has fundamental implication for understanding of basics of fertilization, embryo development and fertility as well as of stem cells biology and cancer. Nowadays, we are facing with a revolution in biological science, due to the adoption of high-throughput technologies, the so-called *–OMICS*, that are able to provide a huge quantity of new data on cell physiological and pathological processes. Although the knowledge of complex phenomena, such as the regulatory mechanisms involved in both germ cell (GC) specification and the maintenance of the germline in adults, is rapidly increasing unfortunately, some aspects of GSCs and of germ cells are still poorly understood. For instance, the biology of male GCs and their signalling machinery still poses important open questions to be answered, as proven by the high incidence of male infertility cases in which it is impossible to reach a diagnosis (unexplained infertility of male origin).

Here, we carried out a review of current information about male GCs biology, with particular respect to their signalling systems located at membrane level.

2. Germline stem cells and hypothalamus-pituitary-testis axis (HPTA)

One of the key events during embryogenesis is the development of germline stem cells, able to originate mature gametes, sperm or oocytes, becoming responsible for transmitting genetic information from generation to generation. In most mammals, such as mice, the germ cell lineage is determined in the early post-implantation embryo, at approximately 3 weeks after fertilization (E17, embryonic day 17). GSCs specification from somatic lineage occurs by appropriate signals from pluripotent embryonic cells (epigenetic mode): a few epiblast cells become competent in response to bone morphogenetic protein (BMP) and wingless-related integration site family of proteins (WNTs) signals produced by extraembryonic ectoderm (ExE) and primitive endoderm (VE). Among the signals responsible for the induction of the germ cell fate, it is possible to distinguish Bmp4 and Bmp8b produced by the ExE, as well as the signal transducers Smad1, 4 and 5. In addition, Bmp2 arisen from the VE seems to improve the role of Bmp4 to ensure the correct production of GSC. These signals induce the expression of the crucial complex of GSC fate, such as BLIMP1 (also known as PRDM1), PRDM14 and AP2γ. These last three factors are able to up-regulate some germ cell genes (such as Stella) and pluripotency genes (OCT4, NANOG and SOX2) and to repress somatic genes (Hoxb1, Hoxa1, Evx1 and Lim1). Soon after specification, GSC migrates through the hindgut and dorsal mesentery, and finally colonizes the genital ridges until E11.5.

During this migratory phase, a special epigenetic remodelling takes place and it includes DNA demethylation, changes of histone modifications, X-chromosome reactivation and genomic imprint erasure. At E13.5, in the gonads, they initiate the sex differentiation either towards a spermatogenic (male) or to an oogenic (female) lineage development [1, 2].

As regards the spermatogenic development, male germline stem cells (also called spermatogonial stem cells, SSCs) enter into mitotic quiescence until the end of foetal development. Soon after birth, SSCs resume active mitotic proliferation at the basement membrane of the seminiferous tubules. Furthermore, SSCs are able to balance self-renewing divisions and differentiating divisions. This delicate balance is also maintained from the complex paracrine dialogue with surrounding somatic microenvironment (stem cell niche) consisting of an ensemble of Sertoli, Leydig, peritubular myoid and vascular cells. This stem cell niche is important not only for self-renewal but also for maintaining stem cells, regulating multipotency, asymmetric cell division and migration from niches for differentiation [3].

During early embryo development, the progression of the testis occurs in a gonadotropin-independent manner and is stimulated by the high levels of AMH (anti-Müllerian hormone) produced by Sertoli cells, so being responsible of the differentiation towards male sexual development of the gonads, with the regression of Müllerian ducts. However, during the second trimester of pregnancy and after birth, the follicle-stimulating hormone (FSH) stimulates the proliferation of Sertoli cells so increasing the secretion of AMH and inhibin B, which will act as a negative regulator of the FSH production. At the same time, Leydig cells, regulated by human chorionic gonadotropin (hCG), secrete androgens, which will be responsible of the acquisition and maintaining of some male sexual characters. The pituitary gland initiates producing luteinizing hormone (LH), which is down-regulated by the testosterone secreted by Leydig cells. During this foetal period, the hypothalamus regulates the secretion of gonadotropin-releasing hormone (GnRH), and so stimulating the pituitary to produce LH and FSH, with a higher balance of LH. At the end of pregnancy, the level of these hormones will decrease due to the direct action of oestrogens produced by the placenta, whereas the levels of testosterone will increase as much as in adult life. After birth, the levels of gonadotropins as well as those of testosterone and AMH decrease to a minimum, reaching the maximum levels 3 months after birth and decreasing again from the sixth month until the puberty.

Throughout the childhood, the HPTA axis allows the proliferation of Sertoli and germ cells, but they remain immature. After this period and around the sixth month, a period of quiescence takes place where Leydig cells are missed, thereby decreasing the levels of testosterone. On the other hand, Sertoli cells still remain active and produce AMH at high levels, typical of 'prepubertal' testis.

Once arrived at puberty, the HPTA starts up again and the male sexual characteristics are developed, acquiring the reproductive capacity. Of high importance is the increase on the levels of gonadotropins and because of that the proliferation of Sertoli cells and the rise of testis volume. The high levels of LH produce the differentiation of Leydig cells as well as the maturation of Sertoli cells, the emergence of blood-testis barrier and a lowering of AMH levels. At this point, germ cells enter meiosis, concluding the spermatogenesis [4]. The most primitive SSCs (A-single cells, A_s) are capable to divide normally forming two new A_s cells (self-renewing division) or with an incomplete cytokinesis forming a pair (A-paired, A_{pr}) of cells connected by an intercellular bridge (differentiating division). Then, the A_{pr} cells continue to divide and generate chains of 4, 8, 16 and (sometimes) 32 cells (aligned cells, A_{al}). Recent studies show that the A_s production by cell division is rather rare and the majority of A_s results from the fragmentation of A_{pr} and A_{al} spermatogonia. From longer chains of A_{al} spermatogonia (8, 16 and 32), classes of spermatogonia progressively differentiated (A_1, A_2, A_3, A_4, In (intermediate) and B) are produced. In comparison with the undifferentiated spermatogonia, those already differentiated divide synchronously and show the presence of heterochromatin. In most animal species, spermatogonia B are the last in suffering mitosis, producing two primary spermatocytes that progressively enter meiosis after the foetal life through all the stages of prophase I (leptotene, zygotene, pachytene and diplotene) and undergo a double meiotic division: the first originates two secondary spermatocytes diploid (2n), while the second leads to the formation of four haploid spermatids. Finally, spermatids undergo a series of cytoplasmic and nuclear changes, known as spermiogenesis. During this last phase, some important processes take place, as the DNA compaction, the loss of cytoplasm and the acrosome and flagellar formation, so leading to the release of mature spermatozoa in the lumen of the seminiferous tubule [5].

The whole process of spermatogenesis is strongly regulated by the hypothalamus-pituitary-testis axis, in such a way that the proper functioning of this axis will be responsible for the quantity and quality of the spermatozoa produced. It is important to note the reliance on the correct running of the endocrine system as well, since it will also influence the reproductive system by releasing the right amount of hormones that will allow the success of the process, as will be described later. Before explaining the endocrine control of the process, the development of this axis will be described from the beginning of the embryo life.

The hypothalamus-pituitary-testis axis initiates its function in the hypothalamus, which along with the hypophysis is the main regulator centre of the reproductive function. The hypothalamus develops from the forebrain, which along with the midbrain and hindbrain is one of the three expansions derived from the neural tube during the brain development of the embryo. After 34 days of conception, it is possible to distinguish inside the diencephalon (originated from the forebrain), a little cavity called third ventricle, whose progress will form the thalamus and it in turn will originate the hypothalamus and the epithalamus. It is located above the pituitary gland and below the thalamus, and it is surrounded by the optic chiasm, lamina terminalis, commissure rostrally, cerebral peduncle and the interpeduncular fossa caudally. The hypothalamus could be equally anatomically divided in three regions, each one with a determined cluster of neurons that carry out a specific function: periventricular zone (with periventricular, suprachiasmatic, paraventricular and arcuate nucleus), medial zone (medial preoptic, anterior hypothalamic, dorsomedial, ventromedial, premammillary, mammillary and posterior hypothalamic nucleus) and lateral zone (lateral preoptic, lateral hypothalamic and supraoptic nucleus).

The hypothalamus is highly connected with the rest of the brain through a really extensive number of fibres whose connections are complex and intricate. Therefore, this region is a key point where nerve signals that came from the central nervous system by afferent fibres will be decoded and transformed into hormonal messages (neuronal hormones) which will arrive by portal circulation to the pituitary gland. It, in turn, will release peptide hormones as a response. The hormone that functionally connects hypothalamus to pituitary gland is known as gonadotropin-releasing hormone (GnRH). It has been identified and described by the Nobel Laureates Roger Guillemin and Andrew V. Schally in 1977 and is constituted by 10 amino acids:

pyroGlu-His-Trp-Ser-Tyr-Gly-Leu-Arg-Pro-Gly-NH_2

GnRH is produced from a 92-amino acid preprohormone in the preoptic area of the hypothalamus by GnRH neurons that originate in the nose and migrate into the brain, where they are scattered throughout the medial septum and hypothalamus and connected by dendrite long over 1 mm. They are regulated by several different afferent neurons and by different neurotransmitters such as norepinephrine, GABA and glutamate.

One of the main regulators of GnRH secretion is Kisspeptin, which acts together with oestrogen, as demonstrated by the finding that Kisspeptin-producing neurons also express oestrogen receptor alpha.

Once secreted in portal bloodstream at the median eminence, GnRH binds its specific receptor, the gonadotropin-releasing hormone receptor (GnRHR), a seven-transmembrane G-protein-coupled receptor, in gonadotrope cells. Here, it activates the beta isoform of phosphoinositide phospholipase C, leading to the calcium mobilization from intracellular stores and to the activation of protein kinase C. Finally, as a result of GnRH stimulation, the pituitary cells synthesize and secrete the gonadotropins LH and FSH.

GnRH activity is deeply connected with the regulation of reproductive activity, thus its concentration is very low during childhood, and strongly increases at puberty. During the adulthood, it regulates several biological processes involved in maintaining of fertility and, in particular, in male it sustains the spermatogenesis via FSH and LH.

The pituitary gland is the second component of the axis involved on the regulation of spermatogenesis. It is an endocrine gland located below the hypothalamus, whose main function is to produce various hormones responsible for the homeostasis of the individual. In this endocrine tissue, it is possible to identify three zones anatomically and embryologically different: adenohypophysis or anterior pituitary, intermediate lobe (present in some species or fused with the anterior pituitary in other species) and neurohypophysis or posterior pituitary [6]. Each zone has its own particular role and cell types with an essential function of hormones secretion, among which should be highlighted the importance of luteinizing hormone and follicle-stimulating hormone, both produced by gonadotrophs cells in the anterior pituitary [7].

LH is a heterodimeric glycoprotein composed by α- and β-subunits (similar to FSH, hCG and to thyroid-stimulating hormone (TSH)). The α-subunits contains 92 amino acids in human and 96 amino acids in almost all other vertebrates and is identical to that of LH, FSH, TSH and hCG. The β-subunit has 120 amino acids and confers its specific biologic to the protein, by interacting with the receptor (LHR). The half-life of LH is about 20 min.

In female, LH is involved in the control of ovarian activity and, mainly, of ovulation. In male, it acts on Leydig cells, stimulating the production of testosterone. This hormone, in turn, regulates the expression of the enzyme 17β-hydroxysteroid dehydrogenase, thus converting androstenedione, produced by the gonads, to testosterone [9] that exerts both endocrine and paracrine activities and then is involved in controlling spermatogenesis.

LH is released in response to a delicate feed-back that involves all the structures of hypothalamus-pituitary-testis axis. When blood concentration of T is lowering, GnRH is released by the hypothalamus, thus stimulating the LH release by pituitary gland. As the level of T increases, it inhibits the release of GnRH and LH consequently.

At the same time, androgens (T, DHT) inhibit monoamine oxidase (MAO) in pineal, leading to the increase in melatonin concentrations. Through a melatonin-induced increase of inhibiting factors (GnIH), the levels of LH and FSH are reduced. T can also be aromatized into oestradiol (E2) to inhibit LH.

FSH is a 35.5-kDa glycoprotein heterodimer, and as LH it consists of two polypeptide units, alpha and beta.

The beta subunit of 111 amino acids (FSH-β) is responsible for the binding with the follicle-stimulating hormone receptor (FSHR). The sugar portion of the hormone is covalently bonded to asparagine and is composed of N-acetylgalactosamine, mannose, N-acetylglucosamine, galactose and sialic acid.

FSH is involved in the control of several functions, such as development, growth, pubertal maturation and reproduction. In both *males* and *females*, it stimulates the maturation of germ cells and, in males, it induces Sertoli cells to secrete androgen-binding proteins (ABPs) and stimulates primary spermatocytes to undergo the first division of meiosis, to form secondary spermatocytes.

Although many aspects of the spermatogenesis remain unclear, the complexity of the process and the necessity of a major regulation, which integrates all the components aforementioned and others that are still being investigated, are obvious. More research is needed in order to conclude the unknown aspects of the whole process that entail the creation of these indispensable cells for the perpetuation of life.

3. Membrane-signalling systems in male germ cells

Once the maturing spermatozoa are released in the lumen of tubuli seminiferi, they progress within rete testis and reach the epididymis. Here, their membrane composition changes [8]. Overall, the lipid remodelling of sperm membrane during the epididymis involves the interaction of male germ cells with epididymal cells, fluid, and with 50–800-nm spherical vesicles present in epididymal lumen, the epididymosomes. They are secreted by principal cells of the epididymis and are involved in the exchange of several kinds of molecules with the sperm membrane [9, 10]. As stated by Rejraji '… it does not seem too farfetched to imagine that epididymosomes (and aposomes in general) could exchange lipids and protein materials with sperm cells, contributing to the formation of structures such as rafts in sperm cells membrane' [11]. In keeping with this idea, in mouse model, it has been found that the epididymosomes membranes are more fluid in the head of the epididymis and that their fluidity gradually decreases in the cauda, while the fluidity of sperm membrane increases as the spermatozoa progress along the epididymal duct [11]. More in detail, it has been found that during the epididymal transit the phosphatidylethanolamine (PE):phosphatidylcholine (PC) ratio does not change, while the concentration of sphingomyelin (SM) increases from 20.9% in caput epididymis to over 29% in cauda epididymis. The cholesterol:phospholipids remain constant and the relative amount of polyunsaturated fatty acids (PUFAs) markedly increase, particularly for 22:5 n-6 and 22:6 n-3. Importantly, the cholesterol concentration changes both in absolute and in relative terms: cholesterol 10–15 mol/spermatozoon: caput 6.9 ± 1.4; cauda 2.4 ± 0.4; cholesterol/phospholipid ratio: caput 0.24 ± 0.04; cauda: 0.289 ± 0.07 [11].

At the end of the epididymal maturation, the spermatozoa membranes have their composition fixed. Human spermatozoa membranes are characterized by high concentrations of ether-linked lipids, of unsaturated fatty acyl groups such as docosahexaenoyl (22:6 chains), and of sphingomyelin. Also present is sulphogalactosylglycerolipid or seminolipid, a spermatozoa-specific lipid, which has been demonstrated to be involved in human gametes interaction, and immediately after ejaculation the ration cholesterol/phospholipid is around 1. Ether-linked lipids are abundant in sperm plasma membranes (PM): glycerophospholipids contain either one alkyl ether group at position sn-1 of glycerol (plasmalogens), or one (at position sn-1) or two alkyl ether groups. Choline and ethanolamine plasmalogens will be involved in modulation of membrane fluidity during capacitation. Indeed, they will act conferring a more densely packed structure to the membranes, compared with diacylglycerophospholipids. Polyunsaturated ethanolamine plasmalogens will take part in the process of membrane fusion, and choline plasmalogens contribute to form non-diffusible membrane regions that confer stability to the membranes.

Immediately after ejaculation, mammalian spermatozoa are virtually unable to fertilize; indeed, they gain their full fertilizing ability only after they reside in female genital tract for hours to weeks, depending on the species, where they complete a process of biochemical and functional maturation known as capacitation. This process has been described for the first time in the early 1950s [12–14] and has been intensively studied by several groups in human and in different animal models. To date, it is widely accepted that it implies deep changes in metabolism of male germ cells and that it involves virtually their whole biochemical machinery. In this context, sperm membrane plays a key role for important and peculiar reasons. As first, sperm membranes are the interface of male gametes with external environment. Male gametes, during spermatogenesis and before ejaculation, male gametes are exposed to different environments (testis, epididymis, male ducts) characterized by the presence of very different chemical components. Each of these factors is able to carry out complex interactions with sperm cells, thus modulating their function. In particular, the interaction with female genital tract is able to drive the process of capacitation by activating or inhibiting specific signal transduction pathways. Then, spermatozoa virtually have no cytosol, thus a great amount of the molecules involved in signalling pathways are localized at the cell membranes level. Consequently, these structures are well organized and highly dynamical, and their architecture and chemical composition change markedly during the process acquisition of fertilizing competence. Finally, the physiological end point of capacitation is the onset of acrosome reaction (AR), which consists in the fusion of outer acrosome membrane (OAM) with the plasma membrane in the anterior of sperm head. In other words, the fertilization is made possible by a fine regulation of inhibiting and activating factor acting at membrane level, able to promote the increase in fusogenicity (i.e. the ability to fuse each other) of PM and OAM avoiding, at the same time, their premature loss.

The pivotal importance of membrane changes during capacitation is the reason why this process has attracted the attention of researchers since its discovery. In particular, on one hand, it could be involved in determining pathological conditions that lead to hypofertility or infertility and, on the other one hand, the control of membranes composition and behaviour during capacitation could have important implication for improving the cryopreservation strategies of male gametes in human and in veterinary andrology.

3.1. Spermatozoa membrane dynamics

The data from several groups, obtained in different animal models (particularly boar), converge in describing a multi-step process [15] that leads to the functional maturation of membranes.

Immediately after ejaculation, the spermatozoa are exposed to a gradually increasing concentration of bicarbonate. This ion acts as an activating factor, stimulating a protein kinase A (PKA)-mediated pathway. In detail, HCO_3^- activates a soluble adenylate cyclase (sAC), leading to an increase in the production of cAMP, which in turn activates PKA [16]. This last event represents an important step because it promotes the activation of several enzymes that are involved in lipid translocation across specific domains of sperm PM (particularly located in the anterior area of sperm head). Here, the segregation of specific classes of lipids in the inner or outer leaflet of plasma membrane [17, 18] has been described. The aminophospholipids, phosphatidylserine (PS) and phosphatidylethanolamine are specifically concentrated in the inner leaflet, while choline phospholipids sphingomyelin and phosphatidylcholine in the outer one. This asymmetry is established and actively maintained by the action of translocating enzymes. Two of them (aminophospholipid translocase, also known as flippase, and floppase) are ATPases, thus working against gradient using ATP as energy source and transferring PS and PE from the outer to the inner lipid leaflet or vice versa, respectively. They are constitutively active in mature spermatozoa and are responsible for maintaining the physiological asymmetry of membranes. A third enzyme, the scramblase, acts as a bi-directional carrier with low specificity for specific classes of lipids, simply moving in both directions (inward and outward) across the membrane following the concentration gradient (it does not require ATP), thus reducing phospholipid asymmetry ('lipid scrambling'). This last event represents a pivotal biological end point because it is believed to be mandatory to allow the cholesterol relocalization [19] and consequent extraction from sperm membrane [20] (**Figure 1**).

Recently, it has been proposed that the capacitation-dependent lipid remodelling of sperm membrane and the apoptotic pathway could be interconnected. In particular, the generation of reactive oxygen species (ROS), particularly peroxynitrite, which takes place during capacitation, could facilitate the removal of cholesterol from PM [21], thus increasing its fluidity, cause a change in the pattern of protein tyrosine phosphorylation and increase the cAMP production [22, 23]. If the fertilization does not occur, the accumulation of ROS could activate the apoptosis via the intrinsic pathway [24]. In a computational biology study, our group implemented this hypothesis, speculating that the spermatozoa, during their journey to reach the fertilizing ability, could pass through an intermediate condition, from which they could reach very different fates: fertilizing spermatozoa, apoptotic spermatozoa, dead spermatozoa. In other words, in earlier stages, it is possible to hypothesize that capacitation and apoptosis are partially overlapping, proceeding parallel, rather than in series [25].

In addition, in spermatozoa, as it occurs in other eukaryotic cell types, specialized micro- and macro-areas known as micro-domains have been described. They can be experimentally isolated by using detergents, such as 0.1% Triton X-100, at 4°C in a discontinuous density gradient, as detergent-resistant membrane (DRM). DRM is organized in a 'lipid-ordered' phase (L_o phase) because of their chemical composition: they are rich in cholesterol, sphingomyelin, gangliosides, phospholipids with saturated long-chain acyl chains, and proteins such as glycosylphosphatidylinositol (GPI)-anchored proteins, caveolin and flotillin. DRM is surrounded by a more fluid portion of membrane organized in a 'liquid-disordered phase' membrane (L_d phase), characterized by higher concentration of unsaturated fatty acids. In this context, the cholesterol plays a pivotal role; indeed its hydroxyl group interacts with the

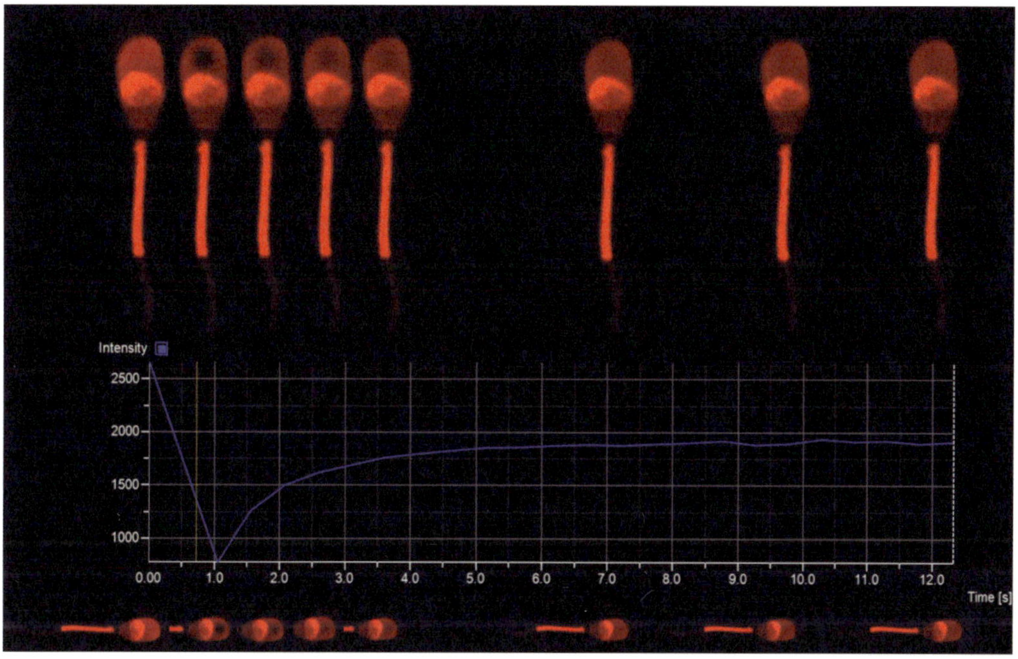

Figure 1. Confocal images of spermatozoa stained with DilC12 probe during a fluorescence recovery after photobleaching (FRAP) experiment, in which it is possible to measure the diffusion coefficient of the probe to assess membrane fluidity.

polar head of phospholipids and sphingolipids, while the steroid and hydrocarbon chains are embedded in the membrane, alongside the nonpolar fatty-acid chain of the other lipids. Consequently, it modulates the physical-chemical proprieties of cell membranes, depending on their composition. In unsaturated fatty acid-rich areas of membrane, cholesterol increases membrane packing, reducing membrane fluidity. On the contrary, when cholesterol intercalates in a microenvironment rich in saturated fatty acids it promotes the relaxation of membrane structure, thus increasing membrane permeability and fusogenicity [18].

DRMs organization undergoes evident modifications, with important physiological consequences on the function of male germ cells. Cross in human spermatozoa described the heterogeneous composition of DRMs and found that the two major raft components, GM1 and CD59, displayed a partial sterol loss-dependent shift to the non-raft domain during capacitation [26]. Miranda et al. demonstrated that LR markers (CAV-2, flotillin 1, flotillin 2 and GM3) changed their immunofluorescence pattern during sperm incubation under capacitating conditions and that these changes are correlated with the occurrence of AR [27]. Watanabe and Kondoh showed that in GFP-labelled sperm, treated with compounds for promoting the acrosome reaction, EGFP-GPI was released from the sperm surface and that ganglioside GM1 relocalizes over sperm head [28]. This leads to hypothesize that GPI-anchored protein release could be associated with reorganization of lipid rafts and with the onset of AR. These data became more interesting when considering that it has been described the capacitation-dependent relocalization in DRMs of proteins known to be involved in signal transduction and in sperm-egg interaction and binding.

For instance, it has been found that cannabinoid receptor type 1 (CB1) and transient receptor potential cation channel subfamily V member 1 (TrpV1) receptors are localized in DRMs at sperm head level. Immediately after ejaculation, CB1 localizes in high-density membrane fractions while, after exposure of spermatozoa to bicarbonate, it redistributes in DRMs. Noteworthy, during this translocation, the glycosylated from of CB1 receptor reaches about 50% of the total molecule. This change suggests that these receptors could play an important role in signalling pathways involved in capacitation [29, 30]. TRPV1 concentration in DRMs increases after exposure to bicarbonate. Since it has been demonstrated that this endocannabinoid-endovanilloid receptor is actively involved in regulation of important biological processes (control of transmembrane potential, regulation of intracellular calcium concentration and actin polymerization) [31, 32], it is possible to hypothesize that its redistribution could have important physiological consequences in controlling the acquisition of fertilizing ability by male germ cells (**Figure 2**).

Similarly, in DRMs, several proteins belonging to the Soluble NSF Attachment Protein REceptor (SNARE) family are present, which are known to be involved in the control of membranes fusion, such as R-SNAREs like synaptobrevin (VAMP) and Q-SNAREs like syntaxin, the Ca^{2+} sensor protein synaptotagmin and the ATPase NSF.

It is very interesting to report that in sperm cells, a protein known to be mainly responsible for the formation of caveolae, caveolin 1 (Cav-1), could be involved in DRMs dynamics without forming caveolae. Travis described the localization of caveolin in rat sperm in cholesterol-enriched areas [33]. This finding led to hypothesizing that this protein could be involved in membrane fusion and, ultimately, AR. Gamboa and Ramalho-Santos in an

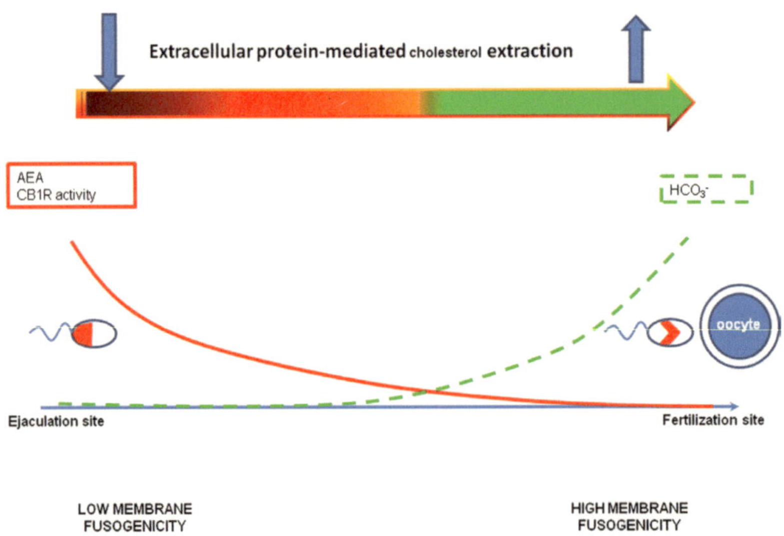

Figure 2. Effect of endocannabinoids and bicarbonate gradients on sperm membrane physico-chemical properties. AEA concentration and CB1R-binding activity decrease (dark gray line) while the bicarbonate concentration increases (light gary dot line). In parallel, the localization of CB1R changes (from Pattern A to Pattern B) and the extracellular protein-mediated cholesterol extraction increases. As a consequence, the membranes became more fusogenic. From Ref. [30].

immunocytochemistry experiment found that anti-Cav-1 antibodies display a strong immunopositivity in acrosomal region and in equatorial segment of the sperm head. Botto et al. (2010) demonstrated that the amount of Cav-1 significantly increases in the insoluble membrane fraction in spermatozoa incubated in vitro under capacitating conditions (from 35 and 20% to 60 and 70%, respectively) when compared with freshly ejaculated sperm cells [34]. More recently, Baltiérrez-Hoyos et al. confirmed the idea that CAV-1 could be involved in biochemical machinery that controls capacitation and the AR. They proposed that it interacts with CDC42, which plays a central role in acrosomal exocytosis through the activation of SNARE proteins and actin polymerization; in particular, they suggested that CDC42 activation is favoured by the disruption of the CAV1–CDC42 interaction [35].

3.2. Membrane fusion and acrosome reaction

The biological end-point of capacitation is the ability to interact with oocyte, undergoing AR. Ultimately, its first step is the fusion of PM and OAM, which is made possible by the lipid remodelling that has occurred during capacitation. The ability of membrane to fuse each other depends on the physical-chemical characteristics of membranes themselves. Indeed, the ability to form 3D structure and the attraction/repulsion between the two membranes vary with the lipid composition of bilayers, and the formation of nucleation points is favoured by the presence of specific families of proteins (fusion proteins). As it is known, from a physical point of view, this event is the result of the coordinated and regulated interplay among various interfacial forces, namely hydration repulsion, hydrophobic attraction and van der Waals forces.

Hydration repulsion: Two hydrated bilayers undergo strong repulsion as they approach each other. This repulsion (hydration repulsion) is due to the water molecules that hydrate the bilayers and is defined as the work required for removing the water molecules bound to hydrophilic molecules exposed to the outside of the bilayer, such as the polar heads of lipids.

The potential V_R is given by

$$V_R = C_R^{[-\frac{z}{\lambda R}]} \tag{1}$$

where C_R (>0) is a measure of the hydration interaction energy for hydrophilic molecules of the given system, λ_R is a characteristic length scale of hydration repulsion, and z is the distance of separation.

Hydrophobic attraction: Hydrophobic force is active attracting two hydrophobic groups in polar media (usually water). In biological membranes, the attractive force between long hydrocarbon chains of lipids represents the main responsible for hydrophobic attraction. The magnitude of this force depends on the hydrophobicity of the interacting molecules and on the distance among them (it decreases approximately exponentially with the distance). This force is the long-ranged and the strongest among all the physical interactions operating between biological surfaces, and it is thought to be involved in folding and stabilization of proteins and macromolecular complexes.

The potential V_A is given by

$$V_A = C_A^{[-\frac{z}{\lambda A}]} \tag{2}$$

where C_A (<0) is a measure of the hydrophobic interaction energy for the given system, λ_A is a characteristic length scale of hydrophobic attraction, and z is the distance of separation.

van der Waals forces: These forces are due to the dipole-dipole interactions (induced/permanent) between the molecules present in membranes. Indeed, as molecules come closer, this attractive force increases due to the ordering of these dipoles.

van der Waals interaction potential $V_{\mathrm{V\,DW}}$ is given by

$$V_{\mathrm{V\,DW}} = \frac{H}{12\,\pi}\left(\frac{1}{z^2} - \frac{2}{(z+2D)^2} + \frac{1}{(z+2D)^2}\right) \tag{3}$$

where H is the Hamaker constant, D and z are the bilayer thickness and the distance of separation, respectively.

The balancing among these forces, as the membranes approach, drives their fusion. In this process, different steps have been identified. First, when the two lipid bilayers became closer, they are weakly attracted by van der Waals forces (that contribute minimally to the evolution of the system) and are subjected by the strong repulsive forces of hydration repulsion. Then, the hydrophobic tails of lipids are exposed to the aqueous phase surrounding them, giving rise to a very strong hydrophobic attraction (which overcomes the repulsive force).

It is worth noting that the lipid remodelling that occurs during capacitation has important implication on the ability of membranes to fuse (membrane fusogenicity). In particular, the chemistry of lipids has a key role in controlling the fusogenicity of membranes. The more the lipid head is polar, the more strongly it binds water and the greater is the hydrophilic repulsion force. On the contrary, the more the lipid acyl chain is longer, the greater is the hydrophobic attraction force. In addition, small polar heads and unsaturation points facilitate the formation of 3D geometries, which is a necessary precondition for membranes fusion.

During capacitation, membranes experience some important changes, which altogether concur in increasing membrane fusogenicity. The lipid scrambling allows the increase of phosphatidylethanolamine, which is characterized by a small slightly polar head, concentration and the increase in unsaturated and PUFA relative concentration (by the cholesterol depletion) in the outer leaflet of PM.

Consequently, at the end of capacitation sperm membranes are fusogenic enough to be able to fuse, but remain unfused waiting for the activator stimulus (the ZP proteins). When the oocyte is met and the spermatozoa interact with ZP, the fusion starts, thanks to the formation of nucleation points, that is, of limited areas where the thermodynamic obstacle of the charges present on membrane surface is overcome. As already told, fusion proteins are the key element of nucleation. In human and animal spermatozoa, the most important fusion proteins are thought to be the SNARE. They are a protein superfamily with more than 60 members that can be divided in two different categories: *vesicle* or *v-SNAREs*, embedded in membranes of transport vesicles, and *target* or *t-SNAREs*, located in the membranes of target compartments. Based on the aminoacidic sequence, they can also be divided in R-SNAREs (arginine-containing SNAREs) or Q-SNAREs (glutamine-containing SNAREs). The SNARE domain is constituted by heptad repeats of 60 amino acids forming a coiled coil.

The mechanism by which SNAREs are involved in membrane fusion is called 'SNARE hypothesis'. This model has been developed in neurons, in which in response to Ca^{2+} influx, synaptic vesicles of neurotransmitter fuse with the membrane at the presynaptic level. The result of vesicle and cell membrane fusion is the release of neurotransmitter into the synaptic cleft. Three different proteins belonging to the SNARE family are involved in this exocytotic event. Vesicle-associated membrane protein (VAMP)-2, located in the vesicular membrane, synaptosome-associated protein (SNAP)-25, which contains two SNARE domains and a region of palmitoylated cysteines, and syntaxin 1A, located in the plasma membrane. At the time of membrane fusion, the coiled-coil-forming domains of syntaxin, SNAP-25 and VAMP form a complex, resistant to sodium dodecyl sulphate (SDS) denaturation, protease digestion and clostridial neurotoxin cleavage, heat stable up to ~90°C. The core of this complex is formed by a long (12-nm), twisted, parallel four-helix bundle: two helices are contributed by SNAP-25 and the others are from VAMP-2 and from syntaxin 1A, respectively. The coiled bundle is 16 layers deep and a layer near the middle, the ionic central layer (the 'zero layer'), contains three glutamines and one arginine (from VAMP-2).

From the data on neuronal SNAREs, a general model has been hypothesized [36, 37]. In the first step, v-SNAREs, on vesicle membrane, form a highly stable trans-complex with t-SNAREs, on cell membrane. The formation of SNARE complex allows the membrane fusion, acting as nucleation point (minimal fusion machinery hypothesis). Interestingly, it is thought that SNAREs have a complex role that go beyond the merely mechanical action. Indeed, they cause the membrane dehydration, thus removing this thermodynamic barrier to fusion, and exert a force on membrane, allowing the formation of a fusion intermediate. After the fusion is completed, SNAREs form a cis-SNARE complex.

The SNARE model of fusion has been proposed also in male [38]. Interestingly, since in spermatozoa AR is a terminal event that occurs only once in cell life, different from what happens in secreting cells where the complex could be disassembled and recycled for further rounds of fusion, here the SNAREs are associated to form ternary cis-complex unstable and insensitive to neurotoxins. When AR takes place, calmodulin is activated by calcium intracellular concentration peak [39] and promotes the activation of RAB3A, which in turn allows the cis-SNAREs disassembly by SF/a-SNAP. Then, monomeric SNAREs form trans-complexes, causing the irreversible docking of the acrosome to the PM. When Ca^{2+} is released from the acrosome through inositol 1,4,5 trisphosphate-sensitive Ca^{2+} channels, the final steps of membrane fusion take place, with the formation of trans-complexes.

Interestingly, in stallion spermatozoa, it has been found that SNARE protein colocalizes with Cav-1 and that fertility seems to be related with the percentage spermatozoa immunopositive for synaptotagmin (a calcium sensor), NSF (a SNARE complex disassembler) and caveolin-1 (a signalling pathways organizer) [34].

4. Cytoskeleton dynamics

During the capacitation, as already told, the membranes fluidity and fusogenicity markedly increase, thus they become more and more instable. This condition on one hand is a prerequisite mandatory to achieve membrane fusion, but on the other one, it could cause the loss of acrosome integrity, with irreversible consequences on fertilizing ability of the gamete. This is the reason why a mechanism that acts as a controller of membrane fusion has been evolved, in sperm head. In this context, the key role is played by actin cytoskeleton. Actin is a 42-kDa protein with a diameter of 4–7 nm present in virtually all the tissues. It has a globular structure, composed by two distinct domains (one larger and one smaller) separated by a cleft, which represents the 'ATPase fold', the centre of enzymatic catalysis that binds ATP and Mg^{2+} and hydrolyses the former to ADP plus phosphate. The domains are separated in subdomains: the smaller domain is composed by subdomain I (lower position, residues 1–32, 70–144 and 338–374) and subdomain II (upper position, residues 33–69). The larger domain is also divided in subdomain III (lower, residues 145–180 and 270–337) and subdomain IV (higher, residues 181–269). What is very important, for the functional characterization of actin polymerization, is that the exposed areas of subdomains I and III form the 'barbed' ends, while the exposed areas of domains II and IV form the 'pointed' ends. The two ends show different affinity for other actin molecules, thus allowing a controlled growth of actin filaments. Indeed, when actin binds ATP forms a stable monomer. Three or more monomers, binding each other, form oligomers that act as nucleation point for the growth of F-actin polymer. Interestingly, unlike other biologically relevant polymers, the monomers of actin are assembled to form filaments by weaker bonds, due to the lateral bonds with neighbouring monomers, which contribute to the stabilization of F-actin. In addition, several proteins are involved in favouring actin polymerization, stabilization and de-polymerization, giving rise to a dynamic process that allows a finely regulated participation of cytoskeleton at a myriad of biological processes.

In spermatozoa, during capacitation G-actin present in sperm head and tail undergoes polymerization under the control of a network of signals. In particular, recent observations suggest that PKA activates Src to inactivate by phosphorylation PIP2-bound gelsolin [40]. Gelsolin is an 82-kD protein with six homologous subdomains (S1–S6), each is composed of a five-stranded β-sheet, flanked by two α-helices. It is one of the members of the actin-severing gelsolin/villin superfamily and acts as a binding protein that regulates actin filament assembly and disassembly. In particular, gelsolin activity is under calcium control and binds to the barbed ends of actin filaments, preventing monomer exchange (end-blocking or capping). In addition, it can promote nucleation (the assembly of monomers into filaments), as well as sever existing filaments. PIP2 is a cofactor for PLD activation stimulated by PKCα, that leads to phosphatidylcholine hydrolysis and production of phosphatidic acid, PA [41, 42]. PA, in turn, activates the polymerization of G-actin to form F-actin. Thus, the activation of PLD and the prevention of F-actin dispersion by inhibiting gelsolin allow F-actin formation. F-actin in the head acts as a diaphragm between PM and OAM, thus preventing immature acrosome reaction. At the AR, the fast peak of intracellular calcium concentration caused the rapid

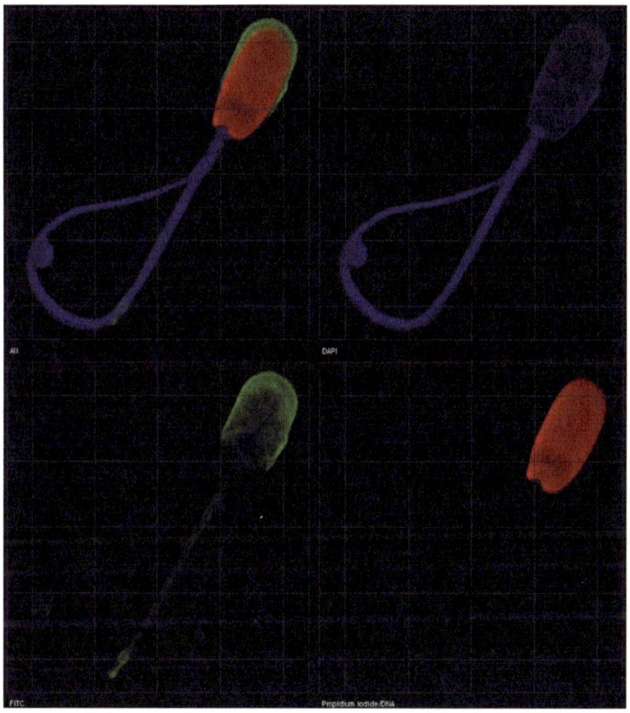

Figure 3. Confocal images showing nucleus (upper right panel), acrosome (lower left panel) and actin cytoskeleton (lower right panel).

destruction of this network, allowing membrane fusion. In the tail, F-actin is thought to play a role in regulating sperm motility including HA motility [40] (**Figure 3**).

Interestingly, actin cytoskeleton has been found to be involved in DRM's stability and relocalization in several cellular models. In spermatozoa, it was observed to move out of the DRM fractions in capacitated sperm [43] and that its polymerization and changes in F-actin structure or orientation during capacitation could be responsible for the loss of association with DRMs [43].

In addition, it has been supposed that F-actin formation during capacitation could have other roles, not merely mechanic, being involved in coordinating the spermatozoa-signalling systems [32]. This suggestion is in keeping with newly emerging evidences that in different cellular systems the cytoskeleton exerts a key role in signal transduction. Indeed, it has been proposed that 'independent of its mechanical strength, the filaments of the cytoskeleton form a continuous, dynamic connection between nearly all cellular structures, and they present an enormous surface area on which proteins and other cytoplasmic components can dock' [44]. This hypothesis is confirmed and strengthened by the finding that in a 20-μm-diameter generic cell the plasma membrane surface area is of about 700 μm^2, while the total surface area of a typical concentration of 10 mg/ml F-actin is 47,000 μm^2 [44] and that the diffusion of signal molecules along cytoskeleton could be a reliable alternative way of intracellular trafficking.

5. GSCs, spermatozoa and endocrine disruptors

The signalling systems that lead GSCs through their road to the differentiation and the achievement of fertilizing ability are very delicate. Any perturbation could cause important negative effects of male fertility. Recently, important international agencies have documented an alarming decrease in human fertility [45, 46]. Although there are yet no conclusive certainties about this phenomenon during the years, different factors have been proposed to be involved in the accumulation of risk factors for infertility and for male infertility. These factors could be either related to social changes as well as to lifestyle [47, 48], such as smoke of tobacco [49–51] and marijuana [52–54], alcohol [55, 56], medications [57] and caffeine [58], but also to the environmental pollution, such as pesticides, solvents [59, 60], electromagnetic fields (EMFs) [61–63] and compounds able to interfere with the endocrine control of biological functions.

One of the most important environmental factors that negatively influence the reproductive health is the exposition to endocrine disruptors, which act altering normal endocrine hormone signalling at the receptor and at the signal transduction level. Exposition to these substances can promote dysfunction in the physiology and epigenetic transgenerational inheritance of disease, affecting also to primordial germ cells. There is a huge number of compounds considered as endocrine disruptors, as, for example, bisphenol A (BPA), vinclozolin (VCZ), dichlorodiphenyltrichloroethane (DDT), methoxychlor, phthalates, genistein, diethylstilbestrol (DES), N,N-diethyl-meta-toluamide (DEET), 2,3,7,8-tetrachlorodibenzo[p]dioxin (TCDD) or jet fuel (JT8).

The study of these disruptors has acquired a higher importance since it has been elucidated that in addition to the direct effects of exposure on an individual these endocrine disruptor compounds (EDCs) are capable of producing also molecular alterations by epigenetic mechanisms, thereby transmitting these changes to the following generations. During the last few years, some researchers have focused their attention on the study of these epigenetic mechanisms, and certain of them will be discussed in order to better understand the *modus operandi* of the participant EDC.

First of all, it is important to note the effects of the widely used bisphenol A, where it is possible to find in many common objects used every day as food containers, feeding bottles or other plastic materials. Some researchers [64] have demonstrated the negative effects of BPA on the expression of pre- and early-meiotic germ cell marker genes and also on somatic cell markers. For example, BPA up-regulates some genes with key roles in germ cell differentiation, as *Stra8* (meiotic entry gene), *Dazl* (required for induction of *Stra8* and initiation of meiosis), *Dmrt1* (gonad-specific transcription factor), *Sycp3* and *Dmc1* (meiosis-specific proteins), modifying also the expression of specific somatic cell markers as *Sox9, Fgf9, Foxl2* and *Wnt4,* and GSC markers as *Oct4, Prdm14* and *Blimp1.*

In relation to plastic materials, the toxic effects of phthalates, plasticizers used to confer flexibility and transparency to these plastic containers, as the di-(2-ethylhexyl) phthalate (DEHP) and the dibutyl phthalate (DBP), whose embryonic exposure was discovered to produce specific changes on the germ cell line [65–67], should also be exposed.

Another EDC that should be mentioned is the fungicide vinclozolin (3-(3, 5-dichlorophenyl)-5-methyl-5-vinyl-oxazolidine-2,4-dione), extensively used in the wine industry and whose metabolites act as antagonists of the androgen receptor (AR)-binding ligand. Many studies [68–70] have been carried out to elucidate the effects of this fungicide, showing how the embryonic exposition to this EDC induces transgenerational defects in spermatogenesis and in sperm viability. Recently, the presence of transgenerational changes in some miRNAs whose target genes are *Lin28/let-7/Blimp1* was discovered, which are involved in the specification of GSCs in mice (also called PGCs, primordial germ cells) [71]. Some phytoestrogens have been also studied by some of the authors, as the isoflavonoids genistein and daidzein, although different results have been obtained by researchers [68, 72] and the mechanism of action and epigenetic modifications should be accurately elucidated yet.

There are many other EDCs commonly used in agriculture as the insecticide dichlorodiphenyltrichloroethane, which has been defined by researchers [73] as promoter of sperm epimutations and differential DNA methylation regions (DMRs) causing transgenerational transmission of obesity. As a substitute of DDT, the pesticide methoxychlor has been used, which is also investigated by some researchers [66, 74] because of the transgenerational defects in sperm induced after embryonic exposure, which confers to the active metabolites the capacity of altering the activity of oestrogens and androgens by a receptor-binding mechanism. Moreover, related to the environmental field it is possible to find the herbicide dioxin (2,3,7,8-tetrachlorodibenzo[p]dioxin), the pesticide permethrin and the insect-repellent N,N-diethyl-meta-toluamide, also studied by researchers [75–77], who concluded their promotion of epigenetic transgenerational inheritance of adult-onset disease.

After the emergence of the idea that maternal exposition during pregnancy to some drugs and chemical compounds was able to produce changes on individual later in life, tributyltin (TBT), an environmental compound able to produce obesity, was studied because of its critical modifications on adipogenesis [78]. In addition to tributyltin, also hydrocarbon mixture of jet fuel was proved to produce epigenetic transgenerational inheritance of disease. This type of hydrocarbon, used by the military, resulted really toxic for the immune system and a promoter of epimutations in sperm in some generations after exposition.

In conclusion, many EDCs have been investigated during the last years. Some of the most important (because of their wide use) have been exposed, but more research is still necessary in order to better understand the new compounds appearing with the new forms of life.

6. Future directions

Nowadays, the extensive adoption of sophisticated biological approaches, such as those based on high-throughput technologies and on *–OMICS*, is providing scientists a huge amount of information. Virtually each month new papers are published about proteomic or genomic and epigenomic analysis of male and female germ cells. This, from one side, could have important positive consequences on our knowledge and on the understanding of human and animal fertility biochemistry and molecular biology, while from the other side poses new problems. The most important one is the so-called big data challenge.

As claimed by authoritative scientists [79, 80], the reductionist paradigm that 'the ultimate aim of the modern movement in biology is to explain all biology in terms of physics and chemistry' [81] is today inadequate to explain complex biological phenomena, as fertility is. The switch from a single molecule-oriented reductionist approach to the whole system-oriented holistic approach (characteristic of systems biology) requires the adoption of mathematical formalisms used in studying complexity. For instance, our group has recently developed a

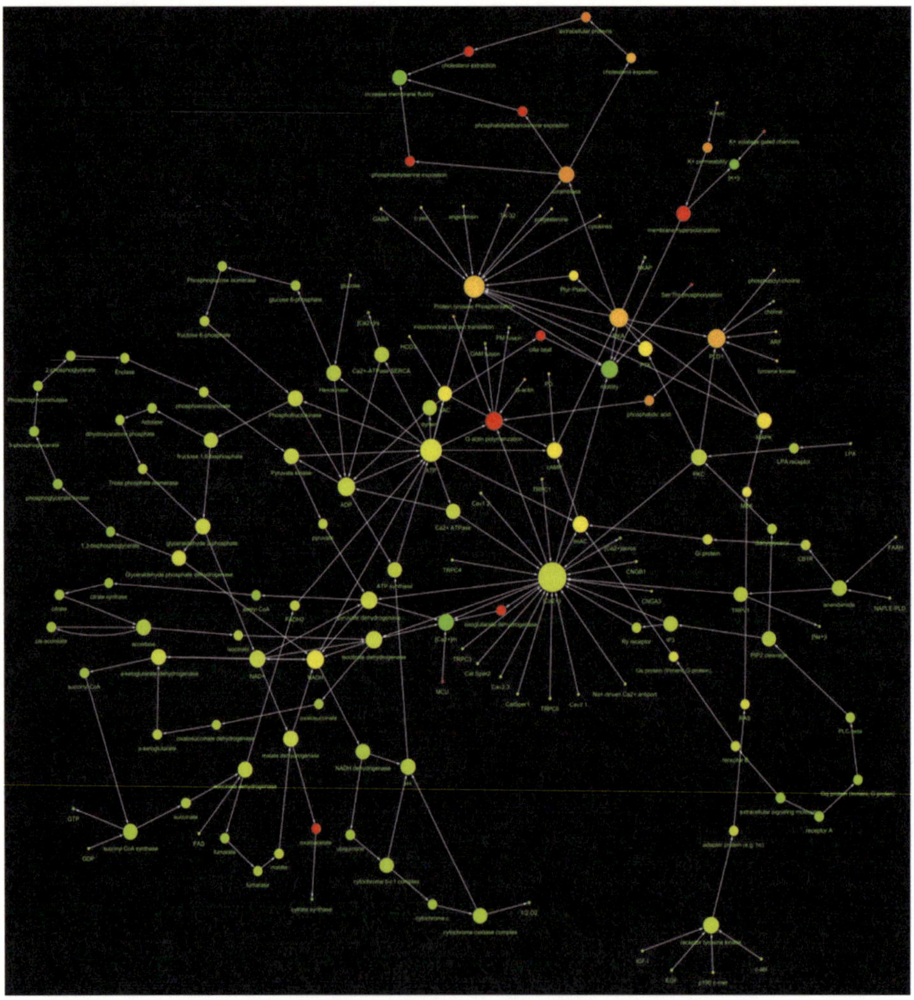

Figure 4. Diagram showing the structure of the capacitation network. The nodes diameter is proportional to the number of links; the gray scale varies depending on the network centrality. The direction of arrows represents the direction of the interaction (from the source to the target). The spatial network arrangement was obtained by using the Cytoscape Spring-embedded Layout (see the text for explanation). From Ref. [83].

biological network-based computational modelling approach, useful to describe and to study the events involved in epididymal maturation of spermatozoa [82], as well as sperm capacitation and acrosome reaction [32, 83–85]. In particular, the molecules involved in these events are represented as nodes linked by their reciprocal interactions, thus originating a network. The analysis of network topology could provide very important information about the architecture of the system and could offer the possibility to take biologically relevant inferences (**Figure 4**).

More in general, in our opinion, one of the most promising directions that are emerging in this fascinating field of research is the adoption of mathematical and computational modelling methods. Obviously, it requires a high degree of interconnection among different disciplines (biology, biochemistry, molecular biology, medical and clinical sciences, computer science, systems science, physics, mathematics and statistics) and it poses new challenges related to the data analysis, data storage and security, data property and data sharing as well as to the availability of computational facilities and resources. But potentially it opens very new and unexpected perspectives on biology of germ cells either in physiological and pathological conditions and could be useful in studying infertility of unexplained origin.

7. Conclusion

The study of GSCs and of CGs is a very fascinating branch of biology that could give information important for basics and applied science and that could contribute in the understanding of infertility causes.

Much has been done and much still remains to be done, here we conclude with the WHO statement '*Advances in our understanding of the signal transduction pathways regulating sperm function will have implications for the development of diagnostic tests capable of generating detailed information on the precise nature of the processes that are defective in the spermatozoa of infertile men*' [86].

Acknowledgements

Marina Ramal Sanchez is granted by the European Union, Horizon 2020 Marie Sklodowska-Curie Action REPBIOTECH 675526.

Abbreviations

WNTs	Wingless-related integration site family of proteins
Smad1 4 5	Small mother against decapentaplegic 1, 4, 5, proteins

BLIMP1	A protein that in humans is encoded by the *PRDM1* gene
PRDM1	PR domain zinc finger protein 1
AP2γ	Activator protein 2γ
OCT4	Octamer-binding transcription factor 4
NANOG	A transcription factor encoded by the *NANOG* gene
SOX2	SRY (sex-determining region Y)-box 2
Stella alias DPPA3	Developmental pluripotency-associated protein 3
Hoxb1	A transcription factor involved in controlling the body plan of an embryo along the cranio-caudal axis
Hoxa1	A transcription factor involved in controlling the body plan of an embryo along the cranio-caudal axis
Evx1	Even-Skipped Homeobox 1
Lim1	Transcription factor in mice that is involved in the control of head structures formation
DNA	Deoxyribonucleic acid
FSH	Follicle-stimulating hormone
LH	Luteinizing hormone
GnRH	Gonadotropin-releasing hormone
HPTA	Hypothalamic-pituitary-testicular axis
TSH	Thyroid-stimulating hormone
TSHR	Thyroid-stimulating hormone receptor
T	Testosterone
DHT	Dihydrotestosterone
cAMP	Cyclic adenosine monophosphate
ROS	Reactive oxygen species
EGFP	Enhanced green fluorescent protein
CAV2	Caveolin 2
GM1	Monosialotetrahexosylganglioside
CDC42	Cell division control protein 42 homologue
SNARE	Soluble NSF Attachment Protein) Receptor
RAB3A	Ras-related protein Rab-3

NSF	N-ethylmaleimide-sensitive factor
PIP2	Phosphatidylinositol 4,5-bisphosphate
PLD	Phospholipase D
PKCα	Protein kinase C alpha

Author details

Nicola Bernabò[1]*, Marina Ramal Sanchez[1], Luca Valbonetti[1], Luana Greco[1], Giulia Capacchietti[1], Mauro Mattioli[1,2] and Barbara Barboni[1]

*Address all correspondence to: nbernabo@unite.it

1 Faculty of Biosciences and Technology for Food, Agriculture and Environment, University of Teramo, Italy

2 Istituto Zooprofilattico Sperimentale 'G. Caporale', Teramo, Italy

References

[1] Tang WWC, Kobayashi T, Irie N, Dietmann S, Surani MA. Specification and epigenetic programming of the human germ line. Nature Review Genetics. Nature Research; 2016 Aug;**17**(10):585-600

[2] Nikolic A, Volarevic V, Armstrong L, Lako M, Stojkovic M. Primordial germ cells: Current knowledge and perspectives. Stem Cells International. Hindawi Publishing Corporation; 2016;**2016**:1-8

[3] Lehmann R. Germline stem cells: Origin and destiny. Cell Stem Cell. NIH Public Access; 2012 Jun;**10**(6):729-739

[4] Rey RA. Mini-puberty and true puberty: Differences in testicular function. Annals in Endocrinology (Paris). 2014 May;**75**(2):58-63

[5] Komeya M, Ogawa T. Spermatogonial stem cells: Progress and prospects. Asian Journal of Andrology. Medknow Publications; 2015;**17**(5):771-775

[6] Lechan RM, Toni R. Functional Anatomy of the Hypothalamus and Pituitary. Endotext. MDText.com, Inc. South Dartmouth (MA); 2000

[7] Flament-Durand J. The hypothalamus: Anatomy and functions. Acta Psychiatrica Belgica. 1980;**80**(4):364-375

[8] Gervasi MG, Visconti PE. Molecular changes and signaling events occurring in spermatozoa during epididymal maturation. Andrology [Internet]. 2017;**5**(2):204-218. Available from: http://doi.wiley.com/10.1111/andr.12320

[9] Sullivan R, Frenette G, Girouard J. Epididymosomes are involved in the acquisition of new sperm proteins during epididymal transit. Asian Journal of Andrology. 2007;**9**(4):483-491

[10] Frenette G, Girouard J, D'Amours O, Allard N, Tessier L, Sullivan R. Characterization of two distinct populations of epididymosomes collected in the intraluminal compartment of the bovine cauda epididymis. Biology of Reproduction [Internet]. 2010;**83**(3):473-480 Available from: http://www.ncbi.nlm.nih.gov/pubmed/20554923

[11] Rejraji H, Sion B, Prensier G, Carreras M, Motta C, Frenoux J-M, et al. Lipid remodeling of murine epididymosomes and spermatozoa during epididymal maturation. Biology of Reproduction [Internet]. 2006;**74**(6):1104-1113. Available from: http://www.ncbi.nlm.nih.gov/pubmed/16510839

[12] Austin C. Observations on the penetration of the sperm in the mammalian egg. Australian Journal of Scientific Research Part B. 1951;**4**(4):581-596

[13] Austin CR. The capacitation of the mammalian sperm. Nature. 1952;**170**(4321):326

[14] Chang MC. Fertilizing capacity of spermatozoa deposited into the fallopian tubes. Nature [Internet]. 1951;**168**(4277):697-698. Available from: http://www.nature.com.ezp-prod1.hul.harvard.edu/nature/journal/v168/n4277/abs/168697b0.html%5Cnhttp://www.nature.com/doifinder/10.1038/168697b0

[15] Gadella BM, Harrison RAP. Capacitation induces cyclic adenosine 3′,5′-monophosphate-dependent, but apoptosis-unrelated, exposure of aminophospholipids at the apical head plasma membrane of boar sperm cells. Biology of Reproduction. 2002;**67**:340-350

[16] Navarrete FA1, García-Vázquez FA, Alvau A, Escoffier J, Krapf D, Sánchez-Cárdenas C, Salicioni AM, Darszon A VP. Biphasic role of calcium in mouse sperm capacitation signaling pathways. Journal of Cellular Physiology. 2015;**230**(8):1758-1769

[17] Leahy T, Gadella BM. New insights into the regulation of cholesterol efflux from the sperm membrane. Asian J Androl. 2015 Jul-Aug;**17**(4):561-567. Available from: http://www.ajandrology.com/preprintarticle.asp?id=153309

[18] Gadella BM, Luna C. Cell biology and functional dynamics of the mammalian sperm surface. Theriogenology [Internet]. 2014;**81**:74-84. Available from: http://dx.doi.org/10.1016/j.theriogenology.2013.09.005

[19] Zerbinati C, Caponecchia L, Puca R, Ciacciarelli M, Salacone P, Sebastianelli A, et al. Mass spectrometry profiling of oxysterols in human sperm identifies 25-hydroxycholesterol as a marker of sperm function. Redox Biology [Internet]. Elsevier B.V.; 2017;**11**(November 2016):111-117. Available from: http://dx.doi.org/10.1016/j.redox.2016.11.008

[20] Boerke A, Brouwers JF, Olkkonen VM, van de Lest CH a, Sostaric E, Schoevers EJ, et al. Involvement of bicarbonate-induced radical signaling in oxysterol formation and sterol depletion of capacitating mammalian sperm during in vitro fertilization. Biology of Reproduction [Internet]. 2013 Jan;**88**(1):21. Available from: http://www.ncbi.nlm.nih.gov/pubmed/23115269 [cited: 25 January 2016]

[21] Gosalvez J, Tvrda E, Agarwal A. Free radical and superoxide reactivity detection in semen quality assessment: Past, present, and future. Journal of Assisted Reproduction and Genetics [Internet]. 2017. Jun;**34**(6):697-707. Available from: http://link.springer.com/10.1007/s10815-017-0912-8

[22] Aitken RJ, Jones KT, Robertson SA. Reactive oxygen species and sperm function—In sickness and in health. Journal of Andrology [Internet]. 2012;**33**(6):1096-1106. Available from: http://www.ncbi.nlm.nih.gov/pubmed/22879525 [cited: 25 January 2016]

[23] Aitken RJ, Baker MA, Nixon B. Are sperm capacitation and apoptosis the opposite ends of a continuum driven by oxidative stress? Asian Journal of Andrology [Internet]. 2015;**17**(4):633-639. Available from: http://www.pubmedcentral.nih.gov/articlerender.fcgi?artid=4492056&tool=pmcentrez&rendertype=abstract [cited: 30 November 2015]

[24] Aitken RJ. The capacitation-apoptosis highway: Oxysterols and mammalian sperm function. Biology of Reproduction [Internet]. 2011 Jul;**85**(1):9-12. Available from: http://www.ncbi.nlm.nih.gov/pubmed/21490245 [cited: 6 January 2016]

[25] Bernabò N, Greco L, Ordinelli A, Mattioli M, Barboni B. Capacitation-related lipid remodeling of mammalian spermatozoa membrane determines the final fate of male gametes: A computational biology study. OMICS [Internet]. 2015 Nov;**19**(11):712-721. Available from: http://www.ncbi.nlm.nih.gov/pubmed/26565605 [cited 18 November 2015]

[26] Cross NL. Reorganization of lipid rafts during capacitation of human sperm. Biology of Reproduction. 2004;**71**(4):1367-1373

[27] Miranda P V, Allaire A, Sosnik J, Visconti PE. Localization of low-density detergent-resistant membrane proteins in intact and acrosome-reacted mouse sperm. Biology of Reproduction. 2009;**80**(5):897-904

[28] Watanabe H, Kondoh G. Mouse sperm undergo GPI-anchored protein release associated with lipid raft reorganization and acrosome reaction to acquire fertility. Journal of Cellular Science [Internet]. 2011;**124**(Pt 15):2573-2581. Available from: http://www.ncbi.nlm.nih.gov/pubmed/21750187%5Cnhttp://jcs.biologists.org/content/124/15/2573.full.pdf

[29] Botto L, Bernabò N, Palestini P, Barboni B. Bicarbonate induces membrane reorganization and CBR1 and TRPV1 endocannabinoid receptor migration in lipid microdomains in capacitating boar spermatozoa. Journal of Membrane Biology. 2010;**238**(1-3):33-41

[30] Barboni B, Bernabò N, Palestini P, Botto L, Pistilli MG, Charini M, et al. Type-1 cannabinoid receptors reduce membrane fluidity of capacitated boar sperm by impairing their activation by bicarbonate. PLoS One. 2011;**6**(8):e23038

[31] Bernabò N, Pistilli MG, Mattioli M, Barboni B. Role of TRPV1 channels in boar spermatozoa acquisition of fertilizing ability. Molecular and Cellular Endocrinology [Internet]. 2010 Jul 29;**323**(2):224-231. Available from: http://www.ncbi.nlm.nih.gov/pubmed/20219627 [cited: 4 December 2014]

[32] Bernabò N, Berardinelli P, Mauro A, Russo V, Lucidi P, Mattioli M, et al. The role of actin in capacitation-related signaling: An in silico and in vitro study. BMC Systems Biology. 2011;**5**:47

[33] Travis AJ, Merdiushev T, Vargas LA, Jones BH, Purdon MA, Nipper RW, et al. Expression and localization of caveolin-1, and the presence of membrane rafts, in mouse and Guinea pig spermatozoa. Developmental Biology. 2001;**240**(2):599-610

[34] Gamboa S, Ramalho-Santos J. SNARE proteins and caveolin-1 in stallion spermatozoa: Possible implications for fertility. Theriogenology. 2005;**64**(2):275-291

[35] Baltierrez-Hoyos R, Roa-Espitia AL, Hernandez-Gonzalez EO. The association between CDC42 and caveolin-1 is involved in the regulation of capacitation and acrosome reaction of guinea pig and mouse sperm. Reproduction. 2012;**144**(1):123-134

[36] Han J, Pluhackova K, Böckmann RA. The multifaceted role of SNARE proteins in membrane fusion. Frontiers in Physiology [Internet]. 2017;**8**(January). Available from: http://journal.frontiersin.org/article/10.3389/fphys.2017.00005/full

[37] Kiessling V, Liang B, Kreutzberger AJB, Tamm LK. Planar supported membranes with mobile SNARE proteins and quantitative fluorescence microscopy assays to study synaptic vesicle fusion. Frontiers in Molecular Neuroscience [Internet]. 2017;**10**(March):1-8. Available from: http://journal.frontiersin.org/article/10.3389/fnmol.2017.00072/full

[38] De Blas GA, Roggero CM, Tomes CN, Mayorga LS. Dynamics of SNARE assembly and disassembly during sperm acrosomal exocytosis. PLoS Biology. 2005;**3**(10)

[39] Vicente-Carrillo A, Álvarez-Rodríguez M, Rodríguez-Martínez H. The CatSper channel modulates boar sperm motility during capacitation. Reproductive Biology [Internet]. Society for Biology of Reproduction and the Institute of Animal Reproduction and Food Research of Polish Academy of Sciences in Olsztyn. 2017;(2016):20-24. Available from: http://www.ncbi.nlm.nih.gov/pubmed/28077244%0Ahttp://linkinghub.elsevier.com/retrieve/pii/S1642431X1630081X

[40] Finkelstein M, Etkovitz N, Breitbart H. Role and regulation of sperm gelsolin prior to fertilization. Journal of Biological Chemistry. 2010;**285**(51):39702-39709

[41] Breitbart H, Rotman T, Rubinstein S, Etkovitz N. Role and regulation of PI3K in sperm capacitation and the acrosome reaction. Molecular and Cellular Endocrinology [Internet]. 2010;**314**(2):234-238 Available from: http://dx.doi.org/10.1038/aja.2010.78

[42] Finkelstein M, Megnagi B, Ickowicz D, Breitbart H. Regulation of sperm motility by PIP2(4,5) and actin polymerization. Developmental Biology [Internet]. Elsevier. 2013;**381**(1):62-72. Available from: http://dx.doi.org/10.1016/j.ydbio.2013.06.014

[43] Catherine T, Monzy Thomas RJR. Reorganization of mouse sperm lipid rafts by capacitation. Molecular Reproduction and Development. 2006;**73**:1541-1549

[44] Janmey PA. The cytoskeleton and cell signaling: Component localization and mechanical coupling. Physiological Review [Internet]. 1998;**78**(3):763-781. Available from: http://physrev.physiology.org/content/78/3/763.abstract

[45] Department of Economic and Social Affairs. World fertility report: Fertility at the extremes. 2013. pp. 1-81

[46] Union E. Demography Report—Short Analytical Web Note [Internet]. European Commission. 2015. p. 54. Available from: http://ec.europa.eu/eurostat/documents/3217494/6917833/KE-BM-15-003-EN-N.pdf/76dac490-9176-47bc-80d9-029e1d967af6

[47] Dondorp W, De Wert G, Pennings G, Shenfield F, Devroey P, Tarlatzis B, et al. Lifestyle-related factors and access to medically assisted reproduction. Human Reproduction. 2010;**25**(3):578-583

[48] Alvarez S. Do some addictions interfere with fertility? Fertilily and Sterility [Internet]. Elsevier Inc.; 2015;**103**(1):22-26. Available from: http://dx.doi.org/10.1016/j.fertnstert.2014.11.008

[49] Practice T, Medicine R. Smoking and infertility: A committee opinion. Fertility and Sterility [Internet]. American Society for Reproductive Medicine; 2012;**98**(6):1400-1406. Available from: http://dx.doi.org/10.1016/j.fertnstert.2012.07.1146

[50] Harlev A, Agarwal A, Gunes SO, Shetty A, du Plessis SS. Smoking and male infertility: An evidence-based review. The World Journal of Men's Health [Internet]. 2015;**33**(3):143-160. Available from: http://synapse.koreamed.org/DOIx.php?id=10.5534/wjmh.2015.33.3.143

[51] Dai J-B, Wang Z-X, Qiao Z-D. The hazardous effects of tobacco smoking on male fertility. Asian Journal of Andrology. 2015;**17**(6):954-960

[52] Park B, McPartland JM, Glass M. Cannabis, cannabinoids and reproduction. Prostaglandins, Leukotrienes, and Essential Fatty Acids. 2004;**70**(2):189-197

[53] du Plessis SS, Agarwal A, Syriac A. Marijuana, phytocannabinoids, the endocannabinoid system, and male fertility. Journal of Assisted Reproduction and Genetics. 2015;**32**(11):1575-1588

[54] Brents LK. Marijuana, the endocannabinoid system and the female reproductive system. Yale Journal of Biology & Medicine. 2016;**89**(2):175-191

[55] Klonoff-Cohen H, Lam-Kruglick P, Gonzalez C. Effects of maternal and paternal alcohol consumption on the success rates of in vitro fertilization and gamete intrafallopian transfer. Fertility and Sterility. 2003;**79**(3):330-339

[56] Wdowiak A, Sulima M, Sadowska M, Bakalczuk G, Bojar I. Alcohol consumption and quality of embryos obtained in programmes of in vitro fertilization. Annals of Agricultural and Environmental Medicine. 2014;**21**(2):450-453

[57] Brezina PR, Yunus FN, Zhao Y. Effects of pharmaceutical medications on male fertility. Journal of Reproduction & Infertility. 2012;**13**(1):3-11

[58] Wesselink AK, Wise LA, Rothman KJ, Hahn KA, Mikkelsen EM, Mahalingaiah S, Hatch EE. Caffeine and caffeinated beverage consumption and fecundability in a preconception cohort. Reproductive Toxicology. 2016;**62**:39-45

[59] Sikka SC, Wang R. Endocrine disruptors and estrogenic effects on male reproductive axis. Asian Journal of Andrology. 2008;**10**(1):134-145

[60] Snijder CA, Te velde E, Roeleveld N, Burdorf A. Occupational exposure to chemical substances and time to pregnancy: A systematic review. Human Reproductive Update. 2012;**18**(3):284-300

[61] Agarwal A, Durairajanayagam D. Are men talking their reproductive health away? Asian Journal of Andrology [Internet]. 2014;**17**(3):433-434. Available from: http://www.ajandrology.com/preprintarticle.asp?id=140963%5Cnhttp://www.ncbi.nlm.nih.gov/pubmed/25432495%5Cnhttp://www.pubmedcentral.nih.gov/articlerender.fcgi?artid=PMC4430942

[62] Zalata A, El-Samanoudy AZ, Shaalan D, El-Baiomy Y, Mostafa T. In vitro effect of cell phone radiation on motility, DNA fragmentation and clusterin gene expression in human sperm. International Journal of Fertility and Sterility. 2015;**9**(1):129-136

[63] Bernabò N, Ciccarelli R, Mattioli M, Barboni B. Effect of non-ionizing electromagnetic fields of anthropic origin on male fertility. Current Chemical Biology [Internet]. 2016;**10**(1):18-31. Available from: http://www.eurekaselect.com/openurl/content.php?genre=article&issn=2212-7968&volume=10&issue=1&spage=18

[64] Aoki T, Takada T. Bisphenol A modulates germ cell differentiation and retinoic acid signaling in mouse ES cells. Reproductive Toxicology. 2012 Nov;**34**(3):463-470

[65] Doyle TJ, Bowman JL, Windell VL, McLean DJ, Kim KH. Transgenerational effects of di-(2-ethylhexyl) phthalate on testicular germ cell associations and spermatogonial stem cells in mice. Biology of Reproduction. Society for the Study of Reproduction; 2013 May;**88**(5):112

[66] Manikkam M, Tracey R, Guerrero-Bosagna C, Skinner MK. Plastics derived endocrine disruptors (BPA, DEHP and DBP) induce epigenetic transgenerational inheritance of obesity, reproductive disease and sperm epimutations. Shioda T, editor. PLoS One. 2013 Jan;**8**(1):e55387

[67] Manikkam M, Guerrero-Bosagna C, Tracey R, Haque MM, Skinner MK. Transgenerational actions of environmental compounds on reproductive disease and identification of epigenetic biomarkers of ancestral exposures. Shioda T, editor. PLoS One. 2012 Feb;**7**(2):e31901

[68] Lehraiki A, Messiaen S, Berges R, Canivenc-Lavier M-C, Auger J, Habert R, et al. Antagonistic effects of gestational dietary exposure to low-dose vinclozolin and genistein on rat fetal germ cell development. Reproductive Toxicology. 2011 May;**31**(4):424-430

[69] Anway MD, Cupp AS, Uzumcu M, Skinner MK. epigenetic transgenerational actions of endocrine disruptors and male fertility. Science (80-). 2005;**308**(5727)

[70] Skinner MK, Guerrero-Bosagna C, Haque MM. Environmentally induced epigenetic transgenerational inheritance of sperm epimutations promote genetic mutations. Epigenetics. Taylor & Francis; 2015;**10**(8):762-771

[71] Brieño-Enríquez MA, García-López J, Cárdenas DB, Guibert S, Cleroux E, Děd L, et al. Exposure to endocrine disruptor induces transgenerational epigenetic deregulation of microRNAs in primordial germ cells. Han JY, editor. PLoS One. 2015 Apr;**10**(4):e0124296

[72] Eustache F, Mondon F, Canivenc-Lavier MC, Lesaffre C, Fulla Y, Berges R, et al. Chronic dietary exposure to a low-dose mixture of genistein and vinclozolin modifies the reproductive axis, testis transcriptome, and fertility. Environmental Health Perspectives. 2009 Aug;**117**(8):1272-1279

[73] Skinner MK, Manikkam M, Tracey R, Guerrero-Bosagna C, Haque M, Nilsson EE. Ancestral dichlorodiphenyltrichloroethane (DDT) exposure promotes epigenetic transgenerational inheritance of obesity. BMC Medicine. BioMed Central; 2013 Oct;**11**:228

[74] Paoloni-Giacobino A. Epigenetic effects of methoxychlor and vinclozolin on male gametes. Vitamins and Hormones. 2014:211-227

[75] Manikkam M, Tracey R, Guerrero-Bosagna C, Skinner MK. Dioxin (TCDD) induces epigenetic transgenerational inheritance of adult onset disease and sperm epimutations. Shioda T, editor. PLoS One. 2012 Sep;**7**(9):e46249

[76] Bruner-Tran KL, Osteen KG. Developmental exposure to TCDD reduces fertility and negatively affects pregnancy outcomes across multiple generations. Reproductive Toxicology. 2011 Apr;**31**(3):344-350

[77] Manikkam M, Tracey R, Guerrero-Bosagna C, Skinner MK. Pesticide and insect repellent mixture (permethrin and DEET) induces epigenetic transgenerational inheritance of disease and sperm epimutations. Reproductive Toxicology. NIH Public Access; 2012 Dec;**34**(4):708-719

[78] Chamorro-García R, Sahu M, Abbey RJ, Laude J, Pham N, Blumberg B. Transgenerational inheritance of increased fat depot size, stem cell reprogramming, and hepatic steatosis elicited by prenatal exposure to the obesogen tributyltin in mice. Environmental Health Perspectives. EMBO Rep. 2013 Jan;**121**(3):359-366

[79] Van Regenmortel MHV. Reductionism and complexity scientists now have the tools to unravel biological complexity and overcome the limitations of reductionism. EMBO Rep. 2004;**5**(11):6-10

[80] Mazzocchi F. Exceeding the limits of reductionism and determinism using complexity theory. EMBO Rep. 2008 Jan;**9**(1):10-4

[81] Crick F. Of Molecules and Men [Internet]. Washington: University of Washington Press; 1996. p. 99. Available from: https://books.google.com/books/about/Of_Molecules_and_Men.html?id=iZQKAAAACAAJ&pgis=1

[82] Bernabò N, Di Agostino R, Ordinelli A, Mauro Mattioli BB. The maturation of murine spermatozoa membranes within the epididymis, a computational biology perspective. Systems Biology in Reproductive Medicine. 2016 Oct;**62**(5):299-308

[83] Bernabò N, Mattioli M, Barboni B. The spermatozoa caught in the net: The biological networks to study the male gametes post-ejaculatory life. BMC Systems Biology [Internet]. 2010 Jan;**4**:87. Available from: http://www.pubmedcentral.nih.gov/articlerender.fcgi?artid=2905340&tool=pmcentrez&rendertype=abstract

[84] Bernabo N. Computational modeling of spermatozoa signal transduction pathways: Just a computer game or a reliable tool in studying male gametes function? Journal of Computer Science and Systems Biology [Internet]. 2013;**6**(4):194-205. Available from: http://www.omicsonline.org/computational-modeling-of-spermatozoa-signal-transduction-pathways-jcsb.1000117.php?aid=18331 [cited: 4 December 2014]

[85] Bernabò N, Mattioli M, Barbara B. Signal transduction in the activation of spermatozoa compared to other signalling pathways: A biological networks study. Int J Data Min Bioinform. 2015;**12**(1):59-69

[86] Cooper TG, Noonan E, von Eckardstein S, Auger J, Baker HWG, Behre HM, et al. World Health Organization reference values for human semen characteristics. Human Reproductive Update. 2009;**16**(3):231-245

Chapter 5

Challenging the Paradigms on the Origin, Specification and Development of the Female Germ Line in Placental Mammals

Noelia P. Leopardo, Pablo I.F. Inserra and Alfredo D. Vitullo

Additional information is available at the end of the chapter

http://dx.doi.org/10.5772/intechopen.71559

Abstract

Most of our understanding on the origin, specification and development of the female germ line in placental mammals comes from studies in the laboratory mouse. The molecular pathway leading to the development and establishment of the female germ line in mouse has erected as the paradigm for placental mammals. It remains, however, largely unexplored whether the well-established mouse regulatory pathway is a common mechanism to other or all placental mammals. Discrete differences in mammals other than mouse reveal the existence of alternative mechanisms that challenge the currently accepted tenets on the origin and establishment of the mammalian female germinal reserve. Here, we will discuss the mouse framework in the light of emerging discrepancies seen in other placental mammals.

Keywords: placental mammals, primordial germ cells, female germ line development, germinal reserve, ovarian development

1. Introduction

Germ cells are the only cell types capable of transmitting the genetic traits of an individual. They differentiate into spermatozoa and oocytes in adult testis and ovary, respectively, and give rise to a totipotent zygote after fertilization. Germ cells guarantee the perpetuation and diversification of the genetic information across the generations in most multicellular organisms. The developmental pathways that lead to the formation of a highly specialized germ cell are long and complicated, and the molecules that are involved in this process are still a matter of discussion. One extraordinary feature in the germ cell lineage in mammals is the fact that specification occurs far from the gonads, implying a necessary migratory phase after specification. A second feature is their unique capacity to undergo meiosis, in which chromosome recombination generates genetic variation in the haploid gametes [1–4].

Most of our understanding regarding germ cell specification and differentiation in mammals comes from studies in the laboratory mouse. It is widely accepted that specification of primordial germ cells (PGCs) in mouse takes place at a very early stage in development; more precisely, they are thought to be set apart following blastocyst implantation in the proximal epiblast of the gastrulating embryo [2]. So far, however, no lineage tracing study has shown that those early segregated PGCs finally end up in the gonads [5]. Alternatively, it has been proposed that presumptive early specified PGCs in the proximal epiblast are rather a primordial pool of stem cells from which PGCs can be specified later on in development, probably during migration toward the emerging gonad [5]. Both explanations have been raised from mouse embryo studies. Nevertheless, there are some key embryological differences between the mouse and other mammals, especially at the epiblast stage when PGCs are specified. The epiblast of the murine rodent forms a cup-shaped egg cylinder, but most other mammals have a flat disk-like epiblast. Signals from extraembryonic tissues induce germ cell fate in a subset of epiblast cell at a specific position with optimal concentration and timing of signals. As PGC specification largely depends on signals from surrounding tissues, the morphology of the embryo is crucial for dissecting out the mechanisms of germ line establishment in different mammals since tissues surrounding the epiblast in the egg cylinder are not the same in flat-disk embryos [6].

2. The mouse model for primordial germ cell specification

2.1. The egg cylinder

In mouse, the blastocyst implants in the uterus by E4.5. The inner cell mass (ICM) of blastocyst is the source of epiblast cells. The ICM is segregated into epiblast and hypoblast or the primitive endoderm. Epiblast cells are equipotent and give rise to all the somatic and germ cells. During implantation, when the syncytiotrophoblast starts to penetrate the wall of the uterus, the epiblast and hypoblast are physically constrained and form a bilaminar embryo. The internal epiblast cells reorganize from a ball of cells into a cup-shaped epithelium surrounded by hypoblast. Immediately before gastrulation (E6.0 and E6.5), the mouse embryo can be visualized as a thick-walled cup of tissue (the epiblast or embryonic ectoderm), which gives rise to the entire fetus and some of the placental membranes. A second thick-walled cup of tissue (the extraembryonic ectoderm, ExE) placed overturned on the epiblast will give rise to the main part of the placenta. Both cups are enclosed in a thin bag of primitive endoderm-derived visceral endoderm (VE) [2, 7, 8].

The embryonic disk is forced into a complex shape called the 'egg cylinder' in which the anterior and posterior poles of the embryo come in close proximity to each other. Around

E4.5 and E5.5, the ExE arises from the polar trophoectoderm (TE) and makes contact with the underlying epiblast. At E6.5, gastrulation starts with the formation of the primitive streak at the posterior region of the embryo. At E7.5, epiblast cells migrating first through this structure include the PGC precursors, which form the extraembryonic mesoderm [9, 10].

2.2. Mechanism for PGC specification

In mouse, PGCs originate from the most proximal epiblast cells by induction of the ExE and VE. Both extraembryonic tissues surround the epiblast cell of the postimplantation egg cylinder at around E5.0–E6.0. The ExE and VE release the bone morphogenetic protein (BMP) 4, 8b and 2 to instruct a small number of pluripotent proximal epiblast cells to become competent to be PGCs, suppressing a somatic program that is adopted by neighboring cells [11] (**Figure 1**).

Accordingly, BMP4 released from the ExE activates the expression of B-lymphocyte–induced maturation protein 1 (*Blimp1*), also known as PR domain-containing protein 1 (*Prdm1*), at ~E6.25 and PR domain-containing protein 14 (*Prdm14*) at ~E6.5 in a dose-dependent manner [12–16]. *Bmp2* expressed in the proximal VE enhances the same signaling pathway, ensuring that the highest levels of Bmp signaling occur in the most proximal epiblast [11, 13, 16]. Both *Blimp1* and *Prdm14* together with *Tcfap2c* (also known as *Ap2*γ) [17, 18] are required for PGC specification.

Blimp1 protein signal first appears in about 6 cells in the most proximal epiblast at the posterior side of the embryo. Blimp1^{+} cells initially express the *Hox* genes as well as many other genes known to be involved in embryonic development and suppress the expression of genes associated with pluripotency, such as *Sox2*, *Nanog*, and *Zic3*. At around E6.75–E7.0, *Hox* genes are downregulated and Blimp1^{+} cells regain the expression of pluripotency genes [13–15].

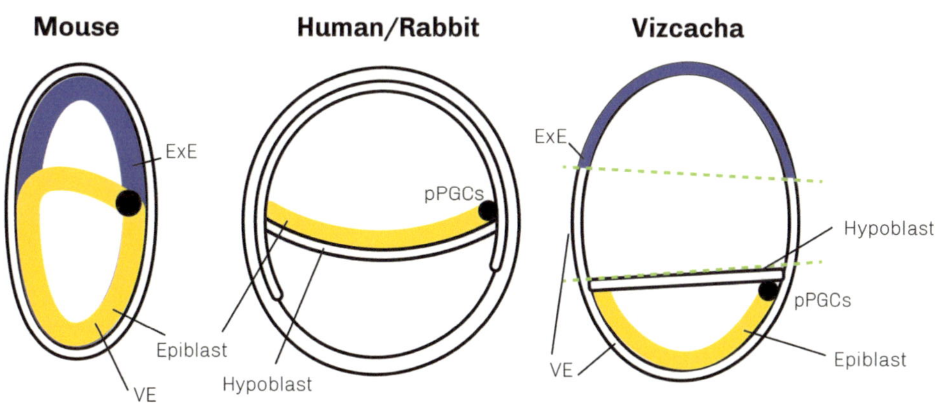

Figure 1. Schematic comparison of the early-implanted embryo in the egg cylinder of mouse and the flat disk embryo of human, rabbit and vizcacha. No extraembryonic ectoderm (ExE) is found in human/rabbit embryo; in the vizcacha, it locates far apart from the epiblast to be responsible for inducing germ cell specification as in mouse. The black circle indicates the presumptive location from which PGCs originate. PGCs: primordial germ cells, pPGC: presumptive PGC, VE: visceral endoderm.

Therefore, the PGC precursors appear to be initially induced toward a somatic mesodermal fate, but then regain their potentially pluripotent nature.

Following lineage restriction, PGC precursors initiate germ cell specification by activating *Prdm14* and *Tcfap2c* [15]. *Prdm14* plays crucial roles in two successive events characterizing the germ cell program: reacquisition of pluripotent potential and epigenetic reprogramming [12, 18]. *Prdm14* is first expressed in Blimp1$^+$ cells and later on in PGCs. Although the activation of *Prdm14* is independent of *Blimp1*, the expression of *Tcfap2c* at ~E6.75 appears to be dependent on *Blimp1* [12]. Indeed, when these factors are coexpressed they can induce PGC-like cells in the absence of cytokines, suggesting that the tripartite gene network *Blimp1/Prdm14 /Tcfap2c* is sufficient for mouse PGC specification [18]. The first two genes acting in the founder PGC population are *Fragilis* and *Stella. Fragilis* (also known as mouse interferon-induced protein like gene-1 [mil-1]/interferon-induced transmembrane protein 3 [*Ifitm3]*) [19] expression marks the beginning of germ cell competence and it starts expressing at ~E6.25–E6.5 before *Blimp1* expression. *Fragilis* expression intensifies in the posterior extraembryonic mesoderm at ~E7.0–E7.25. In fact, the high levels of BMPs activate the expression of *Fragilis* and competent cells acquire the ability to form PGCs when they begin to express *Blimp1*.

Stella (also known as primordial germ cell 7 [Pgc7]/developmental pluripotency-associated 3 [*Dppa3]*) [20] begins to express specifically in *Fragilis-Blimp1* expressing cells in the extraembryonic mesoderm at ~E7.0–E7.25 and continues to be expressed in migrating PGCs. The function of *Stella* gene product is uncertain, but it has domains characteristic of proteins involved in RNA splicing. Actually, *Stella* represses homeobox genes in the nascent germ cell and as such maintains the pluripotency of PGCs during their migration toward the genital ridge. However, gene-knockout studies revealed that neither *Fragilis* nor *Stella* is essential for PGC specification [21, 22].

Blimp$^+$ PGC precursors proliferate and move into the extraembryonic mesoderm (ExM); they reexpress pluripotency-associated genes (*Oct4*, *Nanog*, *Sox2* and *Klf2*) and *Stella* at around E7–E7.75. While Klf2 and Stella are apparently dispensable proteins for PGC development [2, 23], the three core pluripotency factors Oct4, Nanog and Sox2 are essential for PGC development [24–26]. Although the specific roles of these factors during germ cell development are unclear, it is thought that their expression confers latent pluripotency to the germ line. In the case of PGCs, this regulatory network is thought to protect them from somatic-inducing signals during the extensive epigenetic reprogramming they undergo [27]. *Oct4* is uniformly expressed in postimplantation epiblast and also in nascent PGCs during specification. *Oct4* expression remains high until germ cells undergo sexual differentiation in the gonad [28, 29]. It is apparently essential for both germ cell specification [30] and maintenance [31]. *Nanog* is enriched at the proximal posterior epiblast, the position where PGCs are specified from, in E6.5 and E7.5 embryos [32]. *Nanog* appears to be dispensable for mouse PGC specification but is essential for germ cell maintenance. *Sox2* is active in mouse PGC from E7.5 forward. Conditional knockout of *Sox2* shortly after specification caused a dramatic decrease of germ cell numbers by E7.5, being undetectable by E13.5 [32].

With the establishment of germ cell fate, germ cells express factors like alkaline phosphatase (AP), Nanos3, Dazl, mouse vasa homologue (Mvh) and Dnd1 [2]. They increase in number and move out of the embryo by the primitive streak in formation toward the extraembryonic mesoderm at the base of the allantois at E7.25. As mentioned above, PGCs form a cluster of cells 6 to 16 cells at around E6.5; then, they increase to approximately 20–28 cells, move posteriorly and develop into PGCs at E6.75-E7. During early gastrulation, the PGCs form a cluster of 40–50 cells at the base of the incipient allantois in the ExM at around E7.25 [33, 34]. Subsequently, and concomitant with an increase in their number, at around E8, they start to translocate one by one toward the developing hindgut endoderm and move through it. They then leave the endoderm to emerge in the mesentery and at around E10.5 colonize the embryonic gonads, where they proliferate and initiate a differentiation into either oocytes or spermatozoa depending on the embryo sex.

2.3. Migration of PGCs

PGCs in the mouse may be motile from their onset (E7.25) until they colonize the genital ridge (E11.5). After formation, PGCs move through the posterior primitive streak and invade the definitive endoderm and posterior extraembryonic structures. Following subsequent migration within the hindgut during its anterior extension (E8-E9.5), mouse PGCs migrate through the hindgut tissue to the mesoderm, followed by bilateral migration toward the gonadal ridges (E10.5–11.5). During this pregonadic phase, PGCs can be identified by morphological criteria and surface markers, such TNAP and SSEA-1, and the expression of pluripotent markers like Oct4, Sox2 or Nanog [35].

Six distinct stages of PGC behavior in the migratory process were identified, including: (i) invasion of the endoderm, (ii) passive or active migration into the hindgut, (iii) random migration within the hindgut, (iv) migration from the gut to the genital ridges, (v) clustering at the ridges and (vi) cell death within midline structures [36].

At E7.5, PGCs move through the primitive streak and into the definitive endoderm. Some PGCs also end up in the allantois and/or parietal endoderm. The fate of PGCs in extraembryonic structures remains uncertain, but PGCs in the definitive endoderm become incorporated into the hindgut, and at E9.0, they can be found moving within and around the cells of the hindgut epithelium [36]. At E8.5, PGCs on the lip of the hindgut pocket have a rounded non-motile morphology suggesting that PGCs are passively incorporated into the gut and then, at stage (iii), they reinitiate active motility around the epithelial cells.

Interactions between PGCs may also be important for their homing behavior. PGCs emerge from the gut individually, but during migration, they interact with each other forming a migrating network of cells [37]. This network becomes progressively aggregated into clusters of cells toward the end of migration. Antibodies against E-cadherin blocked the process of PGC aggregation in cultured embryo slices and prevented PGCs from forming tight clusters at the genital ridges [38].

At the end of their migration, PGCs presumably lose their motile properties as they associate with somatic cells in the gonad and acquire sex-specific morphologies. There does not seem to be any evidence for sex-specific differences during germ cell migration.

2.4. An alternative hypothesis for PGC specification in mouse

The mouse pathway described above is the classical currently accepted model of PGC formation. This path establishes that PGCs originate and specify as an early lineage-restricted cluster of cells in the base of the allantois soon after implantation. Nevertheless, no definitive proof demonstrating the continuity of those presumptive early-specified PGC and the germ cells, which colonize the genital ridge, has so far been provided. In view of this, and critically reviewing the literature on PGC origin and specification in mouse, Mikedis and Downs [5] advocate in favor of an alternative hypothesis. These authors propose an alternative model in which the presumptive PGCs in the base of the allantois are instead a pool of pluripotent progenitor cells in the posterior end of the primitive streak that builds up the fetal-placental interface. The pluripotent cell pool condenses into a specific area of the proximal epiblast, namely the allantoic core domain (ACD), which extends the body axis posteriorly through the allantoic midline. The pluripotent cells in the ACD express all PGC markers and contribute to both embryonic and extraembryonic tissues. From this pluripotent population, it is suggested that PGC could be segregated later. PGC specification could take place for example during migration toward the genital ridge once evolutionarily conserved genes of germ line development, such as *VASA, Dazl* and *Nanos*, begin to be expressed. Although this alternative explanation is proposed for the mouse egg cylinder, it may well apply in flat embryos where the ExE is absent or far apart from the epiblast.

3. PGC specification and migration in mammals other than the mouse

The embryo proper of most gastrulation-stage mammals, including humans, rabbits and pigs among others, has the shape of a flat disk with two cell layers: epiblast and hypoblast (equivalent to VE in mice) [39–41]. In the flat disk of non-rodent embryos, the epiblast contacts with the VE (hypoblast), and the ExE is absent. In basal rodents of the suborder Hystricognathi such as the guinea pig (*Cavia porcellus*) and the vizcacha (*Lagostomus maximus*), the ExE persists in the flat-disk embryo, but it remains far apart from the epiblast at the time of PGC induction [42, 43]. Moreover, murine PGC nest in the growing mesodermal allantois in the proximal/posterior region of the embryo is a precocious structure found in the mouse, but not seen in nonrodent mammals. These differences have a critical effect on PGC specification factors [4].

3.1. Human

Due to ethical and technical reasons, there is limited information on the origin of human PGCs in postimplantation embryos. PGCs have been described in human embryos at early somite stage in the dorsal wall of the yolk sac near the developing allantois [44–46]. Decades later, AP activity in presumably PGCs was observed by several groups in human embryos with 5–8 somites at a similar location. Using single cell analysis, human PGCs isolated at 4 weeks of development seem to express *PRDM14* and *TFAP2C*, whereas *BLIMP1* and *FRAGILIS* are not expressed [48], suggesting that the critical molecular network in mouse and human early PGCs is divergent. A recent report showed that *BLIMP1* is activated in human PGC-like (hPGCL) cells after specification by *SOX17*, and it is suggested that its role is to inhibit the potential for somatic differentiation [47, 48]. SOX17 is the earliest marker of hPGCL cells and it is in fact the key regulator of their fate, which is not the case in mice. *BLIMP1* is downstream of *SOX17*, and it represses endodermal and other somatic genes. Furthermore, hPGCL cells arise from precursors expressing high levels of *T* and low levels of *SOX2*, resembling posterior primitive streak-derived progenitors [32]. This suggests that human germ cell precursors may arise from a population of posterior primitive streak-derived cells that activate *BLIMP1* in response to paracrine signals, a process that occurs during postgastrulation (later than mice) [34]. The precise combination of signals that promote germ line segregation in humans is currently unknown; however, recent studies in emerging models as cynomolgus macaque, together with *in vitro* studies in human PGC-like cells derived from induced pluripotent stem cells, reveal a different molecular pathway from that evolved in mouse [46].

3.2. Rabbit

In pregastrulation rabbit embryos, *BMP2* is first expressed from the hypoblast and yolk sac epithelium at the boundary of the embryonic disk, which is equivalent to the proximal VE and extraembryonic VE in mice, respectively. In turn, rabbit *BMP4* expression is significantly delayed compared to the mouse. BMP4 marker is first detected during primitive streak formation and it is expressed peripherally in intraembryonic hypoblast and epiblast and in the mesoderm at the posterior pole of the embryonic disk. Interestingly, BLIMP1+ single PGC precursors are detected before primitive streak formation and *BLIMP1* mRNA distribution closely follows the expression pattern of BMP2. Thus, it is proposed that BMP2 may play a more essential role in rabbit PGC specification than BMP4 [49].

On the other hand, PG-2 (a germ cell epitope) and *BLIMP1*-expressing cells have been localized at early gastrulation stage in a region identified in the posterior upper layer (epiblast) and mesoderm [50]. However, *BLIMP1* shows a wider expression pattern during these developmental stages, with positive cells in the hypoblast all around the circumference of the embryo, adjacent to the site of *BMP4* expression in the extraembryonic cells surrounding the embryo. Nevertheless, from these 'blimped' pPGCs, only the posterior ones seem to become PG-2-positive [50].

3.3. Plains vizcacha

A recent study in the basal Hystricognathi rodent *Lagostomus maximus*, which develops through a flat-disk epiblast far apart from the ExE (**Figure 1**), showed that OCT4 protein seems to play an essential role in the establishment and maintenance of the germ line [43]. *OCT4* expression in the pregastrulating embryo was observed across all the epiblast cells, but after the primitive streak stage, *OCT4* was mostly downregulated, and its expression only persisted in a group of cells that was later restricted to the mesoderm of the posterior end of the embryo. It seems likely that *OCT4* expression is required for maintaining pluripotency, helping to epigenetically reprogram cells for PGC development that will be specified at a later stage, probably suppressing expression of genes involved in mesodermal specification [43]. In this model, *BLIMP1* expression has not been detected during early gastrulation or later stages of development (migration and colonization of the genital ridges). It seems likely that *BLIMP1* would not be necessary for the specification of the germ line in the basal rodent *L. maximus*.

In an advanced stage of development, at neural plate stage, in the base of the allantois in the ectoderm and mesoderm after gastrulation, $OCT4^+$ cells become restricted in number to a group of 6–8 cells, and they begin to express *SOX17, STELLA* and *FRAGILIS*. The temporal colocalization of SOX17 and OCT4 proteins in *L. maximus* seems to play a major role in inhibiting somatic genes and maintaining pluripotency instead of the mouse alternative SOX2/OCT4 [51]. During migration through the gut, *SOX17* is downregulated, and its expression is restored in the oogonia after the colonization of the genital ridges.

Then, in the early- and late-head fold stages in mesoderm and endoderm tissues, the expression of *OCT4* and *SOX17* continues but *FRAGILIS* and *STELLA* are downregulated and turned on again during migration. Another notable protein, the germ line marker VASA, was observed early during the translocation of $OCT4^+$ cells to the hindgut. Thereafter, VASA-expressing cells were detected throughout the migration toward the genital ridges. $OCT4^+/VASA^+$ cells sequentially turned on *STELLA* and *FRAGILIS* during migration. Leopardo and Vitullo [43] suggested that *OCT4/STELLA/FRAGILIS*-expressing cells are finally restricted and specified to form PGCs during migration when the evolutionarily conserved germ line marker VASA is expressed.

The spatiotemporal pattern of expression of germ line markers found in *L. maximus* diverges from the currently accepted model on the origin of PGCs as a lineage-restricted cluster of cells in the base of the allantois, specified early just before, or during, gastrulation. In contrast, in this rodent, specification of germ cells seems to occur during migration of a stem cell pool derived from a pluripotent progenitor population within the embryonic axis as proposed by Mikedis and Downs as an alternative pattern of the classical mouse model [5].

4. The assembly of the mammalian ovary after PGC colonization

4.1. Germ cell proliferation in the fetal and postnatal ovary

The number of PGCs that colonize the genital ridges depends on the species. In mice, beginning with 100–145 PGCs at 8 days postconception (dpc), the number increases exponentially up to 15,000–20,000 oogonia per ovary at 15.5 dpc, the time of entry into meiosis and cessation of mitosis [33, 52–56]. A similar pattern of germ cell proliferation was described in rats [57]. In the basal rodent *L. maximus*, approximately 1000 PGCs are detected by the end of migration, rapidly increasing to 55,000 oogonia once fetal ovary colonization is finished; the number continues to increase to reach more than 3×10^6 germ cells by the end of gestation [43, 58]. The limited human data suggest that 1000–2000 colonizing PGCs reach a maximum of approximately $5–6 \times 10^6$ germ cells per ovary at 20 weeks of gestation [59–62].

After a few rounds of mitosis, colonizing PGCs, now referred to as oogonia, cease proliferation and enter a premeiotic phase, with downregulation of pluripotency-associated genes such as *Oct4* and *Lin28* and upregulation of meiotic genes such as *Scp3* [63, 64]. Oogonia entering meiosis, now called oocytes, undergo prophase of the first meiotic division. Just before or early after birth, depending on the species, oocytes in diplotene stage of meiotic prophase I enter a quiescent state known as dictyate, in which they remain arrested, sometimes for years or decades, until just before ovulation [65, 66].

In mice, entry into meiosis seems to be a synchronized event, with no overlapping between mitosis and meiosis. By 17 dpc, mitotic proliferation is finished and all germ cells initiate meiosis [65] entering meiotic prophase in a wave from the anterior to the posterior end of the ovary [64]. However, there is a marked asynchrony of germ cell development in the human ovary. The onset of meiosis occurs by week 11 of gestation [55], but mitosis continues in more peripherally located germ cells for many weeks thereafter, even when primordial follicles begin to form [64, 67]. In the rat, non overlapping mitosis and meiosis of germ cells occurs as in the mouse [68]. However, the basal rodent *L. maximus* shows asynchrony and overlapping of mitotic and meiotic phases of germ cells in a comparable way as humans [58].

The persistence of PGCs or oogonia in the postnatal ovary has been a matter of discussion throughout the twentieth century since Pearl and Schoppe [69] proposed, in 1921, that postnatal oogenesis might occur in the mammalian adult ovary. Three decades later, in an extensive review of the literature of the time, Zuckerman [70] advocated for the absence of oocyte renewal in the mature mammalian ovary, proposing that mammals are born with a finite nonrenewable oocyte pool, a perspective that was widely accepted for more than 50 years generating a useful framework in advancing our knowledge of ovarian dynamics in placental mammals. Nevertheless, this long-held dogma was challenged in 2004 by Tilly's team [71] with the description of a small population of germ line stem cells in the adult ovary of the laboratory mouse. This observation refueled the possibility that neo-oogenesis could take place in the adult ovary of mammals and evidence for and against this possibility has accumulated over the recent years [72]. Although it has not been proved yet that ovarian stem cells may contribute to replenishment of the adult ovary if needed, the persistence of germ line stem cells has been independently proven in the human, mouse and rat models, as well as their ability to be manipulated *in vitro*, and to give rise to offspring following transplantation [73–75].

4.2. Germ cell death in the fetal and postnatal ovary

Death is a prominent feature of mammalian germ line development, with a predictable temporal and spatial pattern. In fetal life, direct germ cell depletion occurs by means of a constitutive massive germ cell death program, referred to as attrition [59, 60, 76–79]. In adult life, germ cell demise is mainly the result of death of the supporting follicular cells, a process known as follicular atresia [64, 76–78].The main mechanism underlying germ cell attrition and follicular atresia requires the activation of a conserved intracellular program of cell death called apoptosis. The execution of the apoptotic program depends on the coordinated action of a group of genes that will activate as a signaling cascade in response to different stimuli. Depending on the source and type of the stimuli, apoptosis can be initiated through an extrinsic pathway, also referred to as the death receptor pathway, which includes the recognition of death ligands to their cell surface receptors [80] or the intrinsic or mitochondrial pathway, which is mainly regulated through the BCL2 protein family whose members are divided into three groups: proapoptotic proteins, antiapoptotic (or prosurvival) proteins and pore-forming proteins [81]. Extrinsic apoptosis molecules are mainly involved in final follicular regression and atresia and corpus luteum regression [82, 83]. *BCL2* gene family executing the intrinsic apoptosis path plays an essential role in the death of the germ cell proper in the antenatal ovary and of granulosa cells during follicular atresia in the adult ovary [84].

The analysis of the spatial and temporal expression of members belonging to the *BCL2* gene family in the mammalian ovary showed that, in general, the expression of proapoptotic genes is continuous throughout prenatal oogenesis, whereas antiapoptotic members are expressed in a time-restricted pattern associated mainly to differentiation and proliferation of the germ cell [85–90]. The enhanced expression of proapoptotic genes such as *BAX* in the face of antiapoptotic members like *BCL2* gives support to the high rate of apoptosis characterizing the mammalian ovary. The involvement of this biased gene balance in determining death or survival of the germ cell has been experimentally supported by showing that *Bcl2*- and *Bax*-knockout mice have decreased or increased primordial follicle reserve, respectively [91, 92].

The causes that determine massive constitutive death of mammalian female germ cells are poorly understood. This massive elimination may avoid the persistence in the ovary of germ cells exhibiting nuclear or mitochondrial chromosomal/genetic defects [93]. Alternatively, death may relate to the exhaustion of germ cells acting as nurse cells to the surviving oocyte pool [94]. Finally, it has been suggested that massive death may enable the appropriate association between germ cells and pregranulosa cells during ovigerous cords or ovarian cyst breakdown, just before primordial follicles begin to form [95]. In any case, the balance between germ cell death and survival seems to be critical to preclude ovarian dysgenesis or premature ovarian failure and to ensure reproductive success.

Germ cell elimination occurs at different points of fetal development. There are three main waves of germ cell death: (i) at prophase and metaphase of proliferating oogonia, (ii) at pachytene of meiotic prophase I oocytes and (iii) at diplotene of meiotic prophase I oocytes [57, 59, 96]. The vast majority of germ cell death occurs during the second and the third waves. Thus, germ cells entering meiosis are particularly susceptible to cell death [55, 60].

In mice, the maximum number of germ cells is registered at the time of entry of primary oocytes into meiotic prophase. However, up to two-thirds of the germ cells are lost before the ovarian reserve is established just after birth [64, 97, 98]. In rats, germ cells proliferate to reach a peak of 64,000 oogonia at 17.5 dpc, but the number of oocytes falls down to about 39,000 at birth and 19,000 at 2 dpc [57, 96]. Humans display a similar dynamics of germ-cell elimination. After the germ cell peak number of 5–6×10⁶ oocytes that occurs at 5 months postconception, there is a dramatic decline in germ cell numbers similar to that seen in mice and rats. By the time of birth, the number of germ cells drops dramatically to 1–2×10⁶ [59, 61, 64, 96] (**Figure 2**).

Moreover, the process of germ-cell apoptosis continues during postnatal life through follicular atresia. In humans, only 300,000 oocytes survive at 7 years postpartum and fewer than 1000 are present in the years just prior to menopause [59, 61, 96].

4.3. Is massive female germ cell demise a constitutive trait for all mammalian species?

Once PGCs have colonized the fetal gonad, the final endowment that will constitute the oocyte reserve seems to depend largely on the balance between cell proliferation and death. Based on the results of germ cell death displayed by mouse, rat and human, it has been widely accepted that massive intraovarian elimination of germ cells is a constitutive attribute of mammalian ovary for the final establishment of the germinal reserve. After a period of high proliferation of colonizing PGCs to reach the maximal oocyte endowment of the species, the activation of the apoptotic pathway generates a point of inflection in the growth curve of the oocyte population that eliminates from 60 to 85% of newly formed oocytes depending on the species [54, 59, 97] (**Figure 2**). The comparable pattern following the elimination of germ cells quantified in mouse, rat and human, together with the recognition that

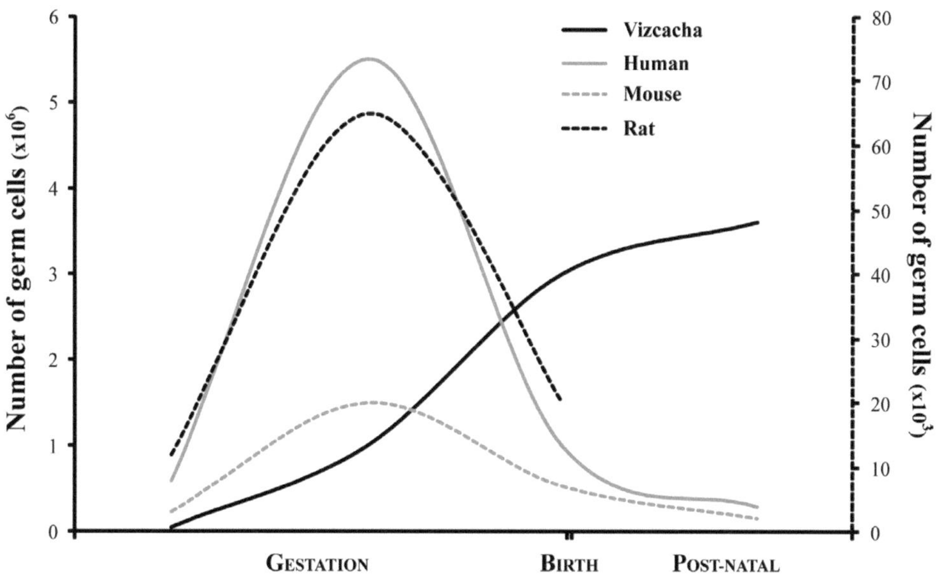

Figure 2. Germ cell growth curves in mammalian species. Human, mouse and rat share the same growth pattern with maximum germ cell endowment at approximately mid-gestation followed by a massive decline through intraovarian cell death. On the contrary, the vizcacha shows a continuous increase of germ cell population, unaffected by cell death.

apoptosis in fetal ovary is active in a few other mammals, proved sufficient to establish massive elimination as a general rule controlling the final oocyte endowment of the ovary in placental mammals.

Challenging this established rule, a quantitative estimate based on unbiased stereological methods showed that the mean germ cell number per ovary increases continuously from the early-developing fetal ovary up to 45–60 days after birth in the South American plains vizcacha, *L. maximus* [58] (**Figure 2**). Female vizcacha displays a constitutive ovary-specific overexpression of the antiapoptotic *BCL2* gene and low to absent expression of proapoptotic *BAX* gene that leads to a strong suppression of apoptosis-dependent germ cell attrition throughout fetal development [99] and apoptosis-dependent follicular atresia throughout adult life [100]. The detection of germ cells undergoing last steps of apoptosis revealed by TUNEL assay never surpasses 4% of the entire germinal population. Hence, the healthy germ cell population increases continuously from early-developing ovary reaching a 50 times higher population number by the end of gestation. Beginning with an endowment of around 56,000 oogonia at 50 dpc, total germ cell number grows up approximately to $3{\times}10^6$ by the end of gestation [58].

Whether the vizcacha is just the exception that confirms the rule or it represents another strategy for establishing the germ cell endowment in mammals, we will have to wait for quantitative studies in a more representative number of placental mammals. Until then, the vizcacha is the first mammal so far described in which female germ line develops in the absence of constitutive massive germ cell elimination since the balance between pro- and anti-apoptotic *BCL2* genes is biased in favor of suppressing apoptosis.

5. Concluding remarks

Our current knowledge regarding the origin and specification of PGCs and the establishment of the ovarian reserve in placental mammals comes by and large from model organisms, notably the mouse. The mouse model has erected as the paradigm for germ line development; however, studies in a few other species unveil differences that challenge the mouse gene network as an established path that may apply to all mammals.

The molecular pathway disclosed for the mouse embryo in the last fifteen years still lacks a final proof showing that the presumptive PGCs, originating early in the proximal epiblast of the egg cylinder, are the same cells that finally colonize the genital ridge later on development. Until this could be traced, alternative hypothesis proposing that PGCs may specify just before colonization from a migrating pluripotent cell population when evolutionarily conserved genes begin to express cannot be ruled out.

The peculiar morphology of the early-implanted mouse embryo, the egg cylinder, sets aside from most mammals that develop through a flat disk embryo. Hence, it is reasonable to suppose that the topographical difference of the gastrulating flat embryo may create a different morphological scenario for signaling and specification of PGCs. The current knowledge in flat embryos, such as those of human and vizcacha, supports a divergent molecular path from that of mouse.

Once the fetal gonad has been colonized by PGCs, it is widely accepted that a balance between proliferation and cell death determines the final oocyte reserve. Massive germ cell death is regarded as an intrinsic shared mechanism in the mammalian ovary regulating the establishment of the final oocyte pool. Nevertheless, only four species have been quantified at the moment and one of these four shows a continuous growth of the germinal population with a minimum cell death. If this is an exception to a general rule or an alternative strategy for establishing the oocyte pool remains unanswered for now.

At this time, we are still far from having a comprehensive knowledge on the possible variety of mechanisms regulating the origin and specification of PGCs and the establishment of the final oocyte reserve in placental mammals. The few species investigated so far seem to indicate that strategies that remain hidden in the great diversity of mammals have not yet been revealed. Comparative studies from different mammalian orders are still lacking and needed.

Abbreviations

PGCs	primordial germ cells
ICM	inner cell mass
ExE	Extraembryonic ectoderm
VE	visceral endoderm
TE	trophoectoderm
ExM	extraembryonic mesoderm
ACD	allantoic core domain
hPGCL	human primordial germ cell-like
pPGC	preprimordial germ cell

Acknowledgements

This study was supported by intramural grant program from Universidad Maimónides-Fundación Científica Felipe Fiorellino and PICT-1281-2014 granted to ADV from the Agencia Nacional de Promoción Científica y Tecnológica, Ministerio de Ciencia, Tecnología e Innovación Productiva, Argentina.

Author details

Noelia P. Leopardo[1,2], Pablo I.F. Inserra[1,2] and Alfredo D. Vitullo[1,2]*

*Address all correspondence to: vitullo.alfredo@maimonides.edu

1 Centro de Estudios Biomédicos, Biotecnológicos, Ambientales y Diagnóstico, CEBBAD-Universidad Maimónides, Buenos Aires, Argentina

2 Consejo Nacional de Investigaciones Científicas y Técnicas, CONICET, Argentina

References

[1] Saitou M, Barton SC, Surani MA. A molecular programme for the specification of germ cell fate in mice. Nature. 2002;**418**:293-300. DOI: 10.1038/nature00927

[2] Irie N, Tang WC, Surani MA. Germ cell specification and pluripotency in mammals: A perspective from early embryogenesis. Reprod Med Biol. 2014;**13**:203-215. DOI: 10.1007/s12522-014-0184-2

[3] Saitou M, Yamaji M. Germ cell specification in mice: Signaling, transcription regulation, and epigenetic consequences. Reproduction. 2010;**139**:931-942. DOI: 10.1530/REP-10-0043

[4] Bertocchini F, Chuva de Sousa Lopes SM. Germline development in amniotes: A paradigm shift in primordial germ cell specification. BioEssays. 2016;**38**:791-800. DOI: 10.1002/bies.201600025

[5] Mikedis MM, Downs KM. Mouse primordial germ cells: A reappraisal. International Review of Cell and Molecular Biology. 2014;**309**:1-57. DOI: 10.1016/B978-0-12-800255-1.00001-6

[6] Sheng G. Epiblast morphogenesis before gastrulation. Developmental Biology. 2015;**401**:17-24. DOI: 10.1016/j.ydbio.2014.10.003

[7] Beddington RS, Robertson EJ. Axis development and early asymmetry in mammals. Cell. 1999;**96**:195-209. DOI: 10.1016/S0092-8674(00)80560-7

[8] Bedzhov I, Zernicka-Goetz M. Self-organizing properties of mouse pluripotent cells initiate morphogenesis upon implantation. Cell. 2014;**156**:1032-1044. DOI: 10.1016/j.cell.2014.01.023

[9] Copp AJ, Cockroft DL, editors. Postimplantation Mammalian Embryos: A Practical Approach. 1st. Oxford: IRL Press-Oxford University Press; 1990. p. 420

[10] Nagy A, Gertsenstein M, Vintersten K, Behringer R, editors. Manipulating the Mouse Embryo: A Laboratory Manual. 3rd. New York: Cold Spring Harbor Laboratory Press; 2003. 100p

[11] Lawson KA, Dunn NR, Roelen BA, Zeinstra LM, Davis AM, Wright CV, Korving JP, Hogan BL. Bmp4 is required for the generation of primordial germ cells in the mouse embryo. Genes & Development. 1999;**13**:424-436

[12] Yamaji M, Seki Y, Kurimoto K, Yabuta Y, Yuasa M, Shigeta M, Yamanaka K, Ohinata Y, Saitou M. Critical function of Prdm14 for the establishment of the germ cell lineage in mice. Nature Genetics. 2008;**40**:1016-1022. DOI: 10.1038/ng.186

[13] Vincent SD, Dunn NR, Sciammas R, Shapiro-Shalef M, Davis MM, Calame K, Bikoff EK, Robertson EJ. The zinc finger transcriptional repressor Blimp1/Prdm1 is dispensable for early axis formation but is required for specification of primordial germ cells in the mouse. Development. 2005;**132**:1315-1325. DOI: 10.1242/dev.01711

[14] Yabuta Y, Kurimoto K, Ohinata Y, Seki Y, Saitou M. Gene expression dynamics during germline specification in mice identified by quantitative single-cell gene expression profiling. Biology of Reproduction. 2006;**75**:705-716. DOI: 10.1095/biolreprod.106.053686

[15] Kurimoto K, Yabuta Y, Ohinata Y, Shigeta M, Yamanaka K, Saitou M. Complex genome-wide transcription dynamics orchestrated by *Blimp1* for the specification of the germ cell lineage in mice. Genes & Development. 2008;**22**:1617-1635. DOI: 10.1101/gad.1649908

[16] Ohinata Y, Payer B, O'Carroll D, Ancelin K, Ono Y, Sano M, Barton SC, Obukhanych T, Nussenzweig M, Tarakhovsky A. *Blimp1* is a critical determinant of the germ cell lineage in mice. Nature. 2005;**436**:207-213. DOI: 10.1038/nature03813

[17] Weber S, Eckert D, Nettersheim D, Gillis AJ, Schafer S, Kuckenberg P, Ehlermann J, Werling U, Biermann K, Looijenga LH. Critical function of AP-2γ/TCFAP2C in mouse embryonic germ cell maintenance. Biology of Reproduction. 2010;**82**:214-223. DOI: 10.1095/biolreprod.109.078717

[18] Magnúsdóttir E, Dietmann S, Murakami K, Günesdogan U, Tang F, Bao S, Diamanti E, Lao K, Gottgens B, Surani AM. A tripartite transcription factor network regulates primordial germ cell specification in mice. Nature Cell Biology. 2013;**15**:905-915. DOI: 10.1038/ncb2798

[19] Tanaka SS, Matsui Y. Developmentally regulated expression of *mil-1* and *mil-2*, mouse interferon-induced transmembrane protein like genes, during formation and differentiation of primordial germ cells. Mechanisms of Development. 2002;**119**:S261-S267

[20] Sato M, Kimura T, Kurokawa K, Fujita Y, Abe K, Masuhara M, Yasunaga T, Ryo A, Yamamoto M, Nakano T. Identification of *PGC7*, a new gene expressed specifically in preimplantation embryos and germ cells. Mechanisms of Development. 2002;**113**:91-94

[21] Payer B, Saitou M, Barton SC, Thresher R, Dixon JP, Zahn D, Colledge WH, Carlton MB, Nakano T, Surani MA. Stella is a maternal effect gene required for normal early development in mice. Current Biology. 2003;**13**:2110-2117

[22] Lange UC, Adams DJ, Lee C, Barton S, Schneider R, Bradley A, Surani MA. Normal germ line establishment in mice carrying a deletion of the *Ifitm/Fragilis* gene family cluster. Molecular and Cellular Biology. 2008;**28**:4688-4696. DOI: 10.1128/MCB.00272-08

[23] Bortvin A, Goodheart M, Liao M, Page DC. Dppa3/Pgc7/stella is a maternal factor and is not required for germ cell specification in mice. BMC Developmental Biology. 2004;**4**:2. DOI: 10.1186/1471-213X-4-2

[24] Kehler J, Tolkunova E, Koschorz B, Pesce M, Gentile L, Boiani M, Lomeli H, Nagy A, McLaughlin KJ, Scholer HR. Oct4 is required for primordial germ cell survival. The EMBO Journal. 2004;**5**:1078-1083. DOI: 10.1038/sj.embor.7400279

[25] Chambers I, Silva J, Colby D, Nichols J, Nijmeijer B, Robertson M, Vrana J, Jones K, Grotewold L, Smith A. Nanog safeguards pluripotency and mediates germline development. Nature. 2007;**450**:1230-1234. DOI: 10.1038/nature06403

[26] Campolo F., Gori M, Favaro R, Nicolis S, Pellegrini M, Botti F, Rossi P, Jannini EA, Dolci S. Essential role of Sox2 for the establishment and maintenance of the germ cell line. Stem Cells. 2013; **31**:1408-1421. DOI: 10.1002/stem.1392l

[27] Leitch HG, Blair K, Mansfield W, Ayetey H, Humphreys P, Nichols J, Surani MA, Smith A. Embryonic germ cells from mice and rats exhibit properties consistent with a generic pluripotent ground state. Development. 2010;**137**:2279-2287. DOI: 10.1242/dev.050427

[28] Yeom YI, Fuhrmann G, Ovitt CE, Brehm A, Ohbo K, Gross M, et al. Germline regulatory element of Oct-4 specific for the totipotent cycle of embryonal cells. Development. 1996;**122**:881-894

[29] Yoshimizu T, Sugiyama N, De Felice M, Yeom YI, Ohbo K, Masuko K, et al. Germline-specific expression of the Oct-4/ green fluorescent protein (GFP) transgene in mice. Development, Growth & Differentiation. 1999;**41**:675-684. DOI: 10.1046/j.1440-169x.1999.00474.x

[30] Okamura D, Tokitake Y, Niwa H, Matsui Y. Requirement of Oct3/4 function for germ cell specification. Developmental Biology. 2008;**317**:576-584. DOI: 10.1016/j.ydbio.2008.03.002

[31] Kehler J, Tolkunova E, Koschorz B, Pesce M, Gentile L, Boiani M. Oct4 is required for primordial germ cell survival. EMBO Reports. 2004;**5**:1078-1083. DOI: 10.1038/sj.embor.7400279

[32] Hart AH, Hartley L, Ibrahim M, Robb L. Identification, cloning and expression analysis of the pluripotency promoting Nanog genes in mouse and human. Developmental Dynamics. 2004;**230**:187-198. DOI: 10.1002/dvdy.20034

[33] Ginsburg M, Snow MH, McLaren A. Primordial germ cells in the mouse embryo during gastrulation. Development. 1990;**110**:521-528

[34] Lawson KA, Hage WJ. Clonal analysis of the origin of primordial germ cells in the mouse. Ciba Foundation Symposium. 1994;**182**:68-84

[35] Oktem O, Oktay K. The ovary. Anatomy and function throughout human life. Annals of the New York Academy of Sciences. 2008;**1127**:1-9. DOI: 10.1196/annals.1434.009

[36] Molyneaux KA, Stallock J, Schaible K, Wylie C. Time-lapse analysis of living mouse germ cell migration. Developmental Biology. 2001;**240**:488-498. DOI: 10.1006/dbio.2001.0436

[37] Anderson R, Fassler R, Georges-Labouesse E, Hynes RO, Bader B l, Kreidberg JA, Schaible K, Heasman J, Wylie C. Mouse primordial germ cells lacking beta1 integrins enter the germline but fail to migrate normally to the gonads. Development. 1999;**126**:1655-1664

[38] Gomperts M, Garcia-Castro M, Wylie C, Heasman J. Interactions between primordial germ cells play a role in their migration in mouse embryos. Development. 1994;**120**:135-141

[39] Flechon JE. Morphological aspects of embryonic disc at the time of its appearance in the blastocyst of farm mammals [Sow, ewe and rabbit, scanning electron microscopy]. Scanning Electron Microscope (USA). 1978;**2**:541-546

[40] Barends PM, Stroband HW, Taverne N, te Kronnie G, Leën MP, Blommers PC. Integrity of the preimplantation pig blastocyst during expansion and loss of polar trophectoderm (Rauber cells) and the morphology of the embryoblast as an indicator for developmental stage. Journal of Reproduction and Fertility 1989;**87**:715-726

[41] Vejlsted M, Du Y, Vajta G, Maddox-Hyttel P. Post-hatching development of the porcine and bovine embryo—Defining criteria for expected development *in vivo* and *in vitro*. Theriogenology. 2006;**65**:153-165. DOI: 10.1016/j.theriogenology.2005.09.021

[42] Chuva de Sousa Lopes SM, Roelen BA. Primordial germ cell specification: the importance of being "blimped". Histology and Histopathology. 2008;**23**:1553-1561. DOI: 10.14670/HH-23.1553

[43] Leopardo NP, Vitullo AD. Early embryonic development and spatiotemporal localization of mammalian primordial germ cell-associated proteins in the basal rodent *Lagostomus maximus*. Scientific Reports. 2017;**7**:594. DOI: 10.1038/s41598-017-00723-6

[44] De Felici M. Origin, migration, and proliferation of human primordial germ cells. In: Coticchio G, Albertini DF, De Santis L, eds. Oogenesis. 1st. London: Springer-Verlag; 2013. p. 19-37

[45] Witschi E. Migration of germ cells of human embryos from the yolk sac to the primitive gonadal folds. Contr Embryol Carnegie Inst. 1948;**209**:67-80

[46] Chen D, Gell JJ, Tao Y, Sosa E, Clark AT. Modeling human infertility with pluripotent stem cells. Stem Cell Research. 2017;**21**:187-192. DOI: 10.1016/j.scr.2017.04.005

[47] de Jong J, Stoop H, Gillis A, van Gurp R, van de Geijn G-J, de Boer M. Differential expression of SOX17 and SOX2 in germ cells and stem cells has biological and clinical implications. The Journal of Pathology 2008;**215**:21-30. DOI: 10.1002/path.2332

[48] Irie N. SOX17 is a critical specifier of human primordial germ cell fate. Cell. 2015;**160**:253-268. DOI: 10.1016/j.cell.2014.12.013

[49] Hopf C, Viebahn C, Püschel B. BMP signals and the transcriptional repressor BLIMP1 during germline segregation in the mammalian embryo. Development Genes and Evolution. 2011;**221**:209-223. DOI: 10.1007/s00427-011-0373-5

[50] Flechon JE. Morphological aspects of embryonic disc at the time of its appearance in the blastocyst of farm mammals [Sow, ewe and rabbit, scanning electron microscopy]. Scanning Electron Microscopy. 1978;**2**:541-546

[51] Aksoy I. Sox transcription factors require selective interactions with Oct4 and specific transactivation functions to mediate reprogramming. Stem Cells. 2013;**12**:2632-2646. DOI: 10.1002/stem.1522

[52] Chiquoine AD. The identification, origin and migration of the primordial germ cells in the mouse embryo. The Anatomical Record. 1954;**118**:135-146

[53] Fujimoto T, Miyayama Y, Futura M. The origin, migration and fine morphology of the human primordial germ cells. The Anatomical Record. 1977;**188**:315-330

[54] Hirshfield AN. Development of follicles in the mammalian ovary. International Review of Cytology. 1991;**124**:43-101

[55] Bendsen E, Byskov AG, Andersen CY, Westergaard LG. Number of germ cells and somatic cells in human fetal ovaries during the first weeks after sex differentiation. Human Reproduction. 2006;**21**:30-35

[56] Myers M, Morgan FH, Liew SH, Zerafa N, Gamage TU, Sarraj M, Cook M, Kapic I, Sutherland A, Scott CL, Strasser A, Findlay JK, Kerr JB, Hutt KJ. PUMA regulates germ cell loss and primordial follicle endowment in mice. Reproduction. 2014;**148**:211-219

[57] Beaumont HM, Mandl AM. A quantitative and cytological study of oogonia and oocytes in the foetal and neonatal rat. Proceedings of the Royal Society of London. Series B: Biological Sciences. 1961;**155**:557-579

[58] Inserra PIF, Leopardo NP, Willis MA, Freysselinard A, Vitullo AD. Quantification of healthy and atretic germ cells and follicles in the developing and post-natal ovary of the South American plains vizcacha, *Lagostomus maximus*: Evidence of continuous rise of the germinal reserve. Reproduction. 2014;**147**:199-209

[59] Baker TG. A quantitative and cytological study of germ cells in human ovaries. Proceedings of the Royal Society of London. Series B: Biological Sciences. 1963;**158**:417-433

[60] Baker TG, Franchi LL. The fine structure of oogonia and oocytes in human ovaries. Journal of Cell Science. 1967;**2**:213-224

[61] Wise PM, Priess J, Kashon ML. Menopause: the aging of multiple pacemakers. Science. 1996;**273**:67-70

[62] Mamsen LS, Lutterodt MC, Andersen EW, Byskov AG, Andersen CY. Germ cell numbers in human embryonic and fetal gonads during the first two trimesters of pregnancy: Analysis of six published studies. Human Reproduction. 2011;**26**:2140-2145

[63] Childs AJ, Kinnell HL, He J, Anderson RA. LIN28 is selectively expressed by primordial and pre-meiotic germ cells in the human fetal ovary. Stem Cells and Development. 2012;**21**:2343-2349

[64] Findlay JK, Hutt KJ, Hickey M, Anderson RA. How is the number of primordial follicles in the ovarian reserve established? Biology of Reproduction. 2015;**93**(5):111,1-111,7

[65] Speed RM. Meiosis in the foetal mouse ovary. I. An analysis at the light microscope level using surface-spreading. Chromosoma. 1982;**85**:427-437

[66] McLaren A. Primordial germ cells in the mouse. Developmental Biology. 2003;**262**:1-15

[67] Fulton N, Martins da Silva SJ, Bayne RAL, Anderson RA. Germ cell proliferation and apoptosis in the developing human ovary. Journal of Clinical Endocrinology and Metabolism. 2005;**90**:4664-4670

[68] Hirshfield AN. Relationship between the supply of primordial follicles and the onset of follicular growth in rats. Biology of Reproduction. 1994;**50**:421-428

[69] Pearl R, Schoppe WF. Studies on the physiology of reproduction in the domestic fowl. The Journal of Experimental Zoology. 1921;**34**:101-111

[70] Zuckerman S. The number of oocytes in the mature ovary. Recent Progress in Hormone Research. 1951;**6**:63-109

[71] Johnson J, Canning J, Kaneko T, Pru JK, Tilly JL. Germline stem cells and follicular renewal in the postnatal mammalian ovary. Nature. 2004;**428**:145-150

[72] Tilly JL, Niikura Y, Rueda BR. The current status of evidence for and against postnatal oogenesis in mammals: A case of ovarian optimism versus pessimism? Biology of Reproduction. 2009;**80**:2-12

[73] Zou K, Hou L, Sun K, Xie W, Wu J. Improved efficiency of female germline stem cell purification using fragilis-based magnetic bead sorting. Stem Cells and Development. 2011;**20**:2197-2204

[74] White YA, Woods DC, Takai Y, Ishihara O, Seki H, Tilly JL. Oocyte formation by mitotically active germ cells purified from ovaries of reproductive-age women. Nature Medicine. 2012;**18**:413-421

[75] Zhou L, Wang L, Kang JX, Xie W, Li X, Wu C, et al. Production of fat-1 transgenic rats using a post-natal female germline stem cell line. Molecular Human Reproduction. 2014;**20**:271-281

[76] Coucouvanis EC, Sherwood SW, Carswell-Crumpton C, Spack EG, Jones PP. Evidence that the mechanism of prenatal germ cell death in the mouse is apoptosis. Experimental Cell Research. 1993;**209**:238-247

[77] De Pol A, Vaccina F, Forabosco A, Cavazzuti E, Marzona L. Apoptosis of germ cells during human prenatal oogenesis. Human Reproduction. 1997;**12**:2235-2241

[78] Kaipia A, Hsueh AJ. Regulation of ovarian follicle atresia. Annual Review of Physiology. 1997;**59**:349-363

[79] Morita Y, Tilly JL. Oocyte apoptosis: Like sand through an hourglass. Developmental Biology. 1999;**213**:1-17

[80] Sheikh MS, Huang Y. Death receptors activation complexes: It takes two to activate TNF receptor 1. Cell Cycle. 2003;**2**:550-552

[81] Willis SN, Adams JM. Life in the balance: How BH3-only proteins induce apoptosis. Current Opinion in Cell Biology. 2005;**17**:617-625

[82] Kondo H, Maruo T, Peng X, Mochizuki M. Immunological evidence for expression of the Fas antigen in the infant and adult human ovary during follicular regression and atresia. The Journal of Clinical Endocrinology and Metabolism. 1996;**81**:2702-2710

[83] Albamonte MS, Albamonte MI, Vitullo AD. Germline apoptosis in the mature human ovary. Journal of Medical Research and Science. 2012;**2**:134-143

[84] Aitken RJ, Findlay JK, Hutt KJ, Kerr JB. Apoptosis in the germ line. Reproduction. 2011;**141**:139-150

[85] De Felici M. Bcl-2 and Bax regulation of apoptosis in germ cell during prenatal oogenesis in the mouse embryo. Cell Death and Differentiation. 1999;**6**:908-915

[86] Kim MR, Tilly JL. Current concepts in Bcl-2 family member regulation of female germ cell development and survival. Biochimica et Biophysica Acta. 2004;**1644**:205-210

[87] De Felici M, Klinger FG, Farini D, Scaldaferri ML, Iona S, Lobascio M. Establishment of oocyte population in the fetal ovary: Primordial germ cell proliferation and oocyte programmed cell death. Reproductive Biomedicine Online. 2005;**10**:182-191

[88] Tilly JL. The molecular basis of ovarian cell death during germ cell attrition, follicular atresia, and luteolysis. Frontiers in Bioscience. 1996;**1**:1-11

[89] Tilly JL, Tilly KI, Perez GI. The genes of cell death and cellular susceptibility to apoptosis in the ovary: A hypothesis. Cell Death and Differentiation. 1997;**4**:180-187

[90] Albamonte MS, Willis MA, Albamonte MI, Jensen F, Espinosa MB, Vitullo AD. The developing human ovary: immunohistochemical analysis of germ-cell specific VASA protein, BCL-2/BAX expression balance and apoptosis. Human Reproduction. 2008;**23**:1895:1901

[91] Knudson CM, Tung KS, Tourtellotte WG, Brown GA, Korsmeyer SJ. Bax-deficient mice with lymphoid hyperplasia and male germ cell death. Science. 1995;**270**:96-99

[92] Ratts VS, Flaws JA, Kolp R, Sorenson CM, Tilly JL. Ablation of bcl-2 gene expression decreases the numbers of oocytes and primordial follicles established in the post-natal female mouse gonad. Endocrinology. 1995;**136**:3665-3668

[93] Tilly JL. Commuting the death sentence: How oocytes strive to survive. Nature Reviews. Molecular Cell Biology. 2001;**2**:838-848

[94] Pepling ME, de Cuevas M, Spradling AC. Germline cysts: A conserved phase of germ cell development? Trends in Cell Biology 1999;**9**:257-262

[95] Guigon CJ, Magre S. Contribution of germ cells to differentiation and maturation of the ovary: Insights from models of germ cell depletion. Biology of Reproduction. 2006;**74**:450-458

[96] Matova N, Cooley L. Comparative aspects of animal oogenesis. Developmental Biology. 2001;**231**(2):291-320

[97] Flaws JA, Hirshfield AN, Hewitt JA, Babus JK, Furth PA. Effect of Bcl-2 on the primordial follicle endowment in the mouse ovary. Biology of Reproduction. 2001;**64**:1153-1159

[98] Kerr JB, Myers M, Britt KL, Mladenovska T, Findlay JK. Quantification of healthy follicles in the neonatal and adult mouse ovary: Evidence for maintenance of primordial follicle supply. Reproduction. 2006;**132**:95-109

[99] Leopardo NP, Jensen F, Willis MA, Espinosa MB, Vitullo AD. The developing ovary of the South American plains vizcacha, *Lagostomus maximus* (Mammalia, Rodentia): Massive proliferation with no sign of apoptosis-mediated germ cell attrition. Reproduction. 2011;**141**:633-641

[100] Jensen FC, Willis MA, Albamonte MS, Espinosa MB, Vitullo AD. Naturally suppressed apoptosis prevents follicular atresia and oocyte reserve decline in the adult ovary of *Lagostomus maximus* (Rodentia, Caviomorpha). Reproduction. 2006;**132**:301-308

Chapter 6

Germ Cell Tumors and their Association with Pregnancy

Mamta Gupta and Vandana Saini

Additional information is available at the end of the chapter

http://dx.doi.org/10.5772/intechopen.72556

Abstract

Ovarian germ cell tumors (OGCTs) comprise 20–25% of all ovarian cancers arising from germ cells of ovary. Mature teratoma (dermoid) is the only benign and commonest germ cell tumor. Only 3–5% germ cell tumors are malignant, dysgerminomas being the most common. These tumors occur in adolescents and reproductive age group. Hence, its association with pregnancy is not uncommon. They can be reliably diagnosed with ultrasound imaging. Raised levels of tumor markers in pregnancy should be interpreted with caution. Cystectomy can be done for benign germ cell tumors. However, fertility sparing surgery with surgical staging with or without adjunctive therapy is recommended for malignant germ cell tumors (MOGTs). Surgery is safe in the second trimester of pregnancy. MOGTs are quite sensitive to chemo and radiotherapy. Three to four courses of chemotherapy with bleomycin, etoposide, and platinum is recommended. Prognosis of these germ cell tumors is excellent.

Keywords: germ cell, germ cell tumors, dermoid cyst in pregnancy, dysgerminoma in pregnancy, immature teratoma, BEP therapy

1. Introduction

Germ cells are the cells in the body that develop into sperms and eggs or oogonia, the gametes. The precursors of germ cells are termed primordial germ cells (PGCs). Like all other somatic cells, the primordial germ cells are diploid. They are present in yolk sac during early embryonic life, and migrate from the yolk sac to its destination, gonadal ridges in the developing gonads. These PGCs proliferate and finally differentiate into oogonia in females. The development and differentiation of PGCs is crucial for assuring normal fertility and the genomic transmission to the next generation [1]. These germ cells are mainly found in the gonads. But, they can sometimes be left behind in other parts of the body during intrauterine development of the individual (extragonadal germ cells).

2. Germ cell tumors

Germ cell tumors (GCTs) are derived from primitive germ cells. More than 90% of GCTs develop in the gonads; ovary or testicle, the remainder is extragonadal, and distributed along the midline of the body, i.e., mediastinum, CNS, retroperitoneum, and sacrococcygeal region [2]. Deregulation of imprinted genes can be associated with tumorigenesis and altered cell differentiation capacity. Ovarian germ cell tumors may be distinguished by their line of differentiation. These tumors can arise from:

1. Primitive totipotent germ cells, i.e., dysgerminoma
2. Primordial germ cells which differentiate into embryonal or extraembryonal cells.
    a. Embryonal cells from which mature and immature teratoma can arise.
    b. Extraembryonal cells i.e., trophoblast and yolk sac from which choriocarcinoma and endodermal sinus tumor can arise respectively.

Ovarian germ cell tumors differ in clinical presentation, histology and biology, and include both benign (predominantly) and malignant subtypes. They constitute about 20–25% of all ovarian neoplasms. Only 5% of germ cell tumors are malignant, with most (95%) being benign mature cystic teratomas. Ovarian malignant germ cell tumors (OMGCTs) include, in order of frequency, dysgerminomas, immature teratomas, yolk sac tumors, and mixed germ cell tumors. Other less common OMGCTs include embryonal carcinomas, choriocarcinomas, and malignant struma ovarii tumors. OMGCTs constitute about 5% of all malignant ovarian neoplasms [3].

A review of the Surveillance, Epidemiology, and End Results (SEER) data taken between 1973 and 2002 reported an incidence of OMGCTs of 3.4/1,000,000 women in the USA [4] and a survey of GCTs in England between 1979 and 2003 [4] reported an incidence of 2.34/1,000,000 women [5]. Data from other countries have reported higher incidence of 5% [3].

The incidence of OGCT is not variable throughout the world. In contrast to epithelial ovarian cancers, there appears to be no racial predisposition; however, incidence of OMGCTs in the Saudi Arabian population (13.8%) was reported approximately three times the incidence of Western populations (5%) and roughly matched the incidence of Asian and African populations (15%) [6].

OMGCTs predominantly occur in young women, but can occur in various other age groups, with the highest incidence in 15–19 years age. The incidence of OGCT increases from the age 8–9 years and peaks at 18 years (20 per million). The mean age of presentation is 19 years. In the first two decades of life, more than 60% of ovarian tumors are of germ cell origin, and one-third of these are malignant. The incidence of OGCT is much lower than testicular tumors; 10.4 per million in females compared to 44.5 per million in males at [7].

3. WHO classification (three categories)

a. Primitive gem cell tumors:

   i. Dysgerminomas

   ii. Nondysgerminomas (yolk sac tumors, embryonal carcinoma, polyembryoma, nongestational carcinoma, and mixed tumors)

b. Biphasic and triphasic germ cell tumors—teratomas

c. Monodermal teratoma and somatic type tumors associated with dermoid cyst

4. Etiology of germ cell tumors

Etiological factors for GCT are ill-understood, apart from an increased incidence associated with dysgenetic gonads. Five percent of patients with dysgerminomas are associated with abnormalities involving the entire or part of the Y chromosome, 46 XY (testicular feminisation), gonadal dysgenesis and mixed gonadal dysgenesis (45 X, 46 XY). However, 95% of females with dysgerminomas are cytogenetically normal [7].

Chromosome 12p abnormalities are frequent in dysgerminoma of the ovary. FISH analysis for chromosome 12p abnormalities may be a used for confirming the diagnosis of dysgerminoma and for differential diagnosis from nongerm cell malignancies [9].

Reduced expression of p16 protein due to INK4A promoter methylation is one of the principal factors that promote cell proliferation in OMGCTs. Thus, p16 may be a novel target for gene therapies to treat OMGCTs [10].

Increased and prolonged expression of stem cell-related proteins (OCT3/4, KIT, and NANOG) in the gonadal tissues of trisomy 21 patients suggests that a delay in fetal germ cell differentiation is a key factor in the development of GCTs [11].

Each of the histological subtype of germ cell cancers show recurrent molecular characteristics of ploidy indices, DNA copy number changes, and specific expression patterns of mRNA, miRNA, and proteins [12].

A familial predisposition has been observed by some with more than one family member or sibling affected. Screening of family members is debatable; however, a discussion regarding these reports with the affected family may be worthwhile [13].

5. Staging of ovarian tumors

Staging of germ cell tumors is as for other ovarian tumors. The FIGO 2014 staging is given in **Table 1** [14].

Stage	Tumor involvement
I	Confined to ovaries
IA	Confined to 1 ovary without capsular/surface involvement, cytology from peritoneal washings or ascitis −ve
IB	Confined to both ovaries without capsular/surface involvement, cytology from peritoneal washings or ascitis −ve
IC	Confined to 1or both ovary with capsular/surface involvement, cytology from peritoneal washings or ascitis +ve
II	Extends beyond ovaries but limited to pelvis
IIA	Extension/implants to uterus/tubes, cytology from peritoneal washings or ascitis −ve
IIB	Extension to other pelvic tissues, cytology from peritoneal washings or ascitis −ve
III	Involves one or both ovaries/fallopian tubes/primary peritoneal cancer, with cytologically or histologically confirmed spread to the peritoneum outside the pelvis and/or metastasis to the retroperitoneal lymph nodes
IIIA	Metastasis to the retroperitoneal LN with or without microscopic peritoneal involvement beyond the pelvis
IIIA1	Positive retroperitoneal lymph nodes only (cytologically or histologically proven)
IIIA2	Microscopic extrapelvic (above the pelvic brim) peritoneal involvement with or without positive retroperitoneal lymph nodes
IIIB	Macroscopic peritoneal metastases beyond the pelvic brim ≤2 cm in greatest dimension, with or without metastasis to the retroperitoneal LN
IIIC	Macroscopic peritoneal metastases beyond the pelvic brim >2 cm in greatest dimension, with or without metastases to the retroperitoneal LN. 1. Includes extension of tumor to capsule of liver and spleen without parenchymal involvement of either organ.
IV	Distant metastases
IVA	Pleural effusion with positive cytology
IVB	Metastases to extra-abdominal organs (including inguinal LN and LN outside abdominal cavity); parenchymal metastases of liver and spleen.

Table 1. FIGO 2014 staging.

6. Germ cell tumors in pregnancy

The incidence of ovarian cancer in pregnancy is quite low, 1 in 12,500–25,000 pregnancies. The estimated incidence of ovarian tumors is approximately 1 in 1000 pregnancies of which approximately 3–6% are malignant [15, 16]. However, a higher incidence of 1 in 143 to 1 in 556 of ovarian tumors in pregnancy has been reported [17, 18]. The incidence of ovarian tumor in pregnant woman requiring surgery was 1 in 1693 (0.025%) [19].

These tumors are relatively asymptomatic; however, the routine use of USG has led to more frequent finding of adnexal masses making diagnosis and management more challenging.

Pregnancy associated with ovarian malignancies present significant challenges and need balancing between optimal maternal therapy and fetal well-being. In addition, cancer diagnosis may be delayed because of difficulties in distinguishing symptomatology from physiologic changes in pregnancy and the difficulty in applying the standard diagnostic work-up in a pregnant woman. Finally, the lack of prospective randomized treatment studies, and therefore, objective data has prevented the development of clinical guidelines for most of the issues complicating the treatment of pregnancy associated ovarian cancer.

6.1. Clinical features

These tumors may be asymptomatic, diagnosed as adnexal mass during routine antenatal ultrasound imaging. The overall estimated incidence of adnexal masses in pregnancy ranges from 2 to 10% [20]. With the use of ultrasound in the first trimester, the reported incidence of adnexal masses has increased. The incidence gradually decreases due to spontaneous resolution of many of these masses as gestation advances. These tumors may present with pain, mass or distension of abdomen, urinary or bowel symptoms. It can be misdiagnosed as fibroid [21]. It can present with acute abdomen, misdiagnosed as acute appendicitis or ectopic pregnancy or with bleeding per vaginum [22]. It is difficult to diagnose ovarian malignancies from functional cysts or benign ovarian tumors. The differentials of such an adnexal mass in pregnancy include ectopic pregnancy, corpus luteal cyst, functional cyst, paraovarian cyst, endometrioma, leiomyoma, and ovarian neoplasms.

6.1.1. Tumor markers in germ cell tumors

The important markers of germ cell tumors are serum alpha feto protein (AFP), human chorionic gonadotropin (hCG), and lactic dehydrogenase (LDH).

Alpha-fetoprotein—it is a normal fetal serum protein synthesized by the liver, yolk sac, and gastrointestinal tract. Almost all endodermal sinus tumors of the ovary express AFP. AFP is also expressed by immature teratomas, ovarian embryonal cell carcinoma, and polyembryomas. It is present in the cytoplasm of tumor cells and in the characteristic hyaline globules observed in the endodermal sinus tumor. It is raised in 85% of patients with these tumors but in only 20% of patients with stage I disease. Hence, this marker has limited role in screening. Typical values seen in normal pregnancy for AFP is 1000 to 10,000 ng/mL, >9 multiples of median [23].

AFP is present in 100% women with yolk sac tumor, 61.9% in immature teratoma, and 11.8% in dysgerminoma, but no positive case for AFP in mature cystic teratoma and mature cystic teratoma with malignant transformation is seen [24].

Pregnancy normal and abnormal, hepatocellular carcinoma, cirrhosis, and hepatitis also may be associated with increased levels of serum AFP. Nevertheless, an extremely raised AFP in a normal pregnancy may be associated with endodermal sinus tumor, an aggressive malignant germ cell tumor.

Human chorionic gonadotropin—it is a glycoprotein produced by syncytiotrophoblast and is made of alpha and beta subunits. Choriocarcinoma gestational and nongestational (ovarian) both express hCG.

LDH-dysgerminomas are commonly associated with elevations in LDH, although it is not elevated in all dysgerminomas. Occasionally, dysgerminomas may become infiltrated with syncytiotrophoblastic giant cells, which produce beta-hCG. Elevations in AFP are less common with dysgerminomas. Many scientists contend that AFP/hCG secreting dysgerminomas are misdiagnosed as pure lesions, and that they actually represent mixed tumors containing other malignant germ cell components.

Mixed lesions may secrete AFP, hCG, or both or neither of these markers, depending on the components.

Therefore, useful tumor markers for the workup of germ cell tumors include-hCG, AFP, LDH, Inhibin A and B to rule out sex cord stromal tumors, Cancer antigen 125 (CA-125) to rule out epithelial tumors.

These serologic elevations of tumor markers readily resolve following surgical excision; and may be used as tumor markers to monitor for recurrence.

6.1.2. Limitation of tumor markers in pregnancy

Some established tumor markers are synthesized and secreted physiologically during fetal development, i.e., hCG, AFP, inhibin, making them less useful during pregnancy [20]. CA125 increases in early pregnancy and post-partum period having limited diagnostic utility. HCG also peaks during the first trimester. The values of tumor markers therefore, should be interpreted with caution during pregnancy and treatment strategies should not be based on levels of these markers alone.

6.2. Imaging

6.2.1. Imaging in malignant and benign tumors

There are numerous ultrasound features of adnexal masses that have been associated with increased risk of malignancy including size, solid components or heterogeneous/complex appearance, excrescences/papillary structures, internal septations, bilaterality, irregular borders, increased vascularity, low resistance blood flow, and presence of ascites [20]. Finding of ascites by ultrasound may be closely related with advanced stage malignancy and bad prognosis [25]. Some germ cell tumors have characteristic imaging features, i.e., dysgerminoma, mature, and immature teratomas can be diagnosed with high accuracy.

MRI may provide additional information. CT is not recommended in pregnancy due to ionization risk to the developing fetus.

6.2.2. Imaging in torsion of tumors

Sonographically ovarian torsion is demonstrated by visualizing an enlarged, edematous ovary along with a mass or cyst. Doppler imaging may fail to demonstrate arterial and/or venous blood flow to the ovary. Ovarian torsion is a clinical diagnosis and ultrasound should only be used to provide additional supportive diagnostic information. A recent study showed that 19% of patients with torsion had normal preoperative Doppler flow to the affected adnexa [26]. The risk of torsion among pregnant patients with adnexal tumors >4 cm increases, 51% of torsions occurred in tumors measuring 6–8 cm in diameter. The highest rate of torsion occurred between 15 and 16 weeks of gestation. Sixty percent of the torsion happened between the 10th and 17th weeks of gestation [27].

6.3. Effect of pregnancy on ovarian tumor

Increased risk of torsion, incarceration, rupture, and hemorrhage can occur during pregnancy and vaginal delivery.

6.4. Effect of ovarian tumors on pregnancy

Spontaneous successful pregnancy with no feto-maternal compromise has been reported [21]. Fetal demise has been reported to be in 25% of cases [28].

6.5. Management in pregnancy

Majority of adnexal masses in pregnancy are benign and a good percentage will spontaneously resolve. About 55% of masses resolve completely or significantly decrease in size [29, 30]. Best predictors of persistence are complex appearance and size greater than 5 cm.

Observation: Patients with simple or functional appearing small adnexal masses should have surveillance with ultrasound every trimester [30, 31].

Surgery: Surgical intervention is required in situations: if malignancy is suspected; if an acute complication, i.e., torsion or rupture develops; if any suspicious mass (complex cyst with solid components or thick septa) more than 5 cm in size persists near 18 weeks, demonstrates a 30–50% increase in size at any time during the pregnancy or exceeds 8 cm in size.

The goals of surgery include: removal of the mass to avoid complications during pregnancy, obtain a diagnosis, and to stage or debulk ovarian cancer if malignancy is identified. Laparotomy for an adnexal mass is done by a midline incision and begins with obtaining peritoneal washings and a complete exploration of the abdomen and contralateral ovary. Manipulation of the uterus should be minimized, as this could increase the risk of placental abruption, premature labor, or fetal loss. If the clinical suspicion for malignancy is low and it seems technically feasible, a cystectomy rather than salpingo-oophorectomy is performed. If, however, the clinical suspicion for cancer is high (excrescences, ascites, etc.) or the mass is solid, the tube and ovary should be removed. In either case, a frozen section should be obtained.

If a malignancy is confirmed and seems to be confined to the ovary, then a full staging surgery including peritoneal biopsies, omentectomy, and lymphadenectomy should be considered; however, the benefit gained from the more extensive surgery must be balanced against potential feto-maternal morbidity. Conservative surgical management for most malignant ovarian germ cell tumors diagnosed during pregnancy should be considered as the proper initial treatment [32]. Staging is critical as adjuvant therapy during pregnancy, is only initiated for those with advanced-stage disease. Routine biopsy or wedge-resection of the contralateral ovary is not necessary unless it seems to be involved with disease.

If metastatic disease is detected, an attempt at cytoreduction should be undertaken. The feto-maternal risk of an extended and radical debulking should be weighed with the potential maternal benefit, realizing that interval cytoreduction after chemotherapy and completion of the pregnancy is a reasonable approach [33]. However, the majority of ovarian cancers associated with pregnancy are diagnosed at an early stage, when disease is still confined to the ovary [34, 35].

In recent years, laparoscopy has been used to manage benign looking adnexal masses with minimal morbidity.

6.6. Timing of intervention

The ideal time for intervention is 14–22 weeks gestational age. It avoids the period of greatest risk of drug-induced teratogenicity; spontaneous fetal losses due to intrinsic fetal abnormalities have already occurred; the function of corpus luteum has been replaced by the placenta; most functional cysts have disappeared; an acceptable operative field is still available, allowing minimal uterine manipulation and low risk of obstetric complications. A later surgery in pregnancy, at the end of second trimester or at third trimester, may be technically more difficult and may result in an adverse obstetric outcome [36].

When indicated for other reasons, cesarean section may also be an opportunity for the surgical management of adnexal masses. In patients who undergo vaginal delivery, and in whom surgery was not indicated antenatally, a repeat imaging should be performed 6–8 weeks post-partum [37].

6.7. Pregnancy outcome after surgical intervention during pregnancy

Surgery is considered safe in second trimester [38] before 23 weeks, yet the decision to proceed with surgical management should outweigh the risks of adverse perinatal outcomes. The incidences of congenital malformations and stillbirths were not increased in the offspring of women having surgery. The incidences of abortions; very-low and low birth weight infants were increased due to increase in the risk of prematurity and intrauterine growth retardation. [39]. The incidence of infants dying within 168 h was increased. No specific types of anesthesia or operation were associated with adverse outcomes [40].

6.8. Oncologic outcome after surgical intervention in pregnancy

Majority of women at the time of diagnosis of ovarian tumors during pregnancy, have favorable results as most have low grade and early stage disease. It is appropriate to consider fertility sparing surgery in these young women. However, there are reports about the rapid growth and recurrence of ovarian germ cell tumors during pregnancy [28]. Hence, patients should undergo comprehensive surgical staging at the time of diagnosis.

6.9. Adjuvant therapy

Germ cell tumors are quite sensitive to chemo and radiotherapy. Chemotherapy usually is the adjuvant of choice to spare fertility. BEP (bleomycin, cisplatin, etoposide) is the standard adjuvant chemotherapy for 3–4 cycles [41]. Recommendations for chemotherapy are:

- Recurrence during observation (for stage IA dysgerminoma and stage IA grade 1 immature teratoma).
- Stage II–IV dysgerminoma.
- Stage II–IV teratoma or stage I grade 2–3.
- Embryonal or endodermal sinus tumor irrespective of stage [42].

6.9.1. Chemotherapy

Chemotherapy should not be given during the first trimester due to high risk of fetal malformations. Fetal congenital malformation risk is 10% for single agent and 25% for combination chemotherapy in first trimester.

Bleomycin—it is a copper-chelating glycoprotein capable of inducing DNA strand scission breaks via oxidative processes. This drug is eliminated by the kidneys. Pulmonary function tests are recommended if bleomycin is considered.

Cisplatin—it inhibits DNA synthesis and, thus, cell proliferation, by causing DNA cross-links and denaturation of the double helix. Cisplatin is excreted by kidneys; those with impaired renal function should postpone therapy.

Carboplatin—carboplatin is an analog of cisplatin. Carboplatin has the same efficacy as cisplatin but with a better toxicity profile. Its main advantages over cisplatin include less nephrotoxicity and ototoxicity not requiring extensive pre-hydration and less likelihood of inducing nausea and vomiting, but it is more likely to induce myelotoxicity.

Etoposide—etoposide inhibits topoisomerase II and causes DNA strand breakage, causing cell proliferation to arrest in the late S or early G2 portion of the cell cycle.

BEP therapy: bleomycin 30 units/week IV on days 1, 8, and 15 plus etoposide 100 mg/m^2/day IV and cisplatin 20 mg/m^2/day IV on days 1 to 5. BEP is given every 21 days for three cycles (or four cycles if the patient had bulky residual disease after surgery).

In women with recurrence, confirmed residual disease, or raised tumor markers after first-line chemotherapy, recommended treatment consists of paclitaxel-ifosfamide-cisplatin (TIP) or another acceptable regimen. TIP is given as follows: paclitaxel 250 mg/m^2 IV infused over 24 h on day 1 plus ifosfamide 1500 mg/m^2/day IV and cisplatin 25 mg/m^2/day IV on days 2 to 6. TIP is given every 21 days for four cycles [42].

6.9.1.1. Complications of chemotherapy

The most common medical complications from chemotherapy are bone marrow abnormalities and renal toxicity. Care should be taken to monitor for signs of pulmonary toxicity in patients receiving bleomycin-containing regimens. Secondary malignancies are rare, but leukemias may occur in patients receiving etoposide, especially if doses exceed 2000 mg/m^2 (i.e., >4 cycles of standard BEP (bleomycin, etoposide, platinum) regimen. BEP treatment has been associated with ventriculomegaly, transient neonatal neutropenia and bilateral sensorineural hearing loss in few cases [43].

6.9.2. Radiation

Loss of fertility is a problem with radiation. Primary therapy with radiation is reserved for patients who are incapable of tolerating chemotherapy or surgical resection. It can be used in stage IB to stage III. Radiation is mostly used to treat periaortic and pelvic lymph node metastases [44].

6.10. Follow up

Recurrence of dysgerminomas is most often seen in the first 2–3 years after treatment. Therefore, follow-up observation and a physical examination every 3–4 months for the first 3 years, every 6 months during the fourth and fifth years, and annual surveillance thereafter is recommended [44].

CT imaging should be considered during months 6 and 12, especially if tumor markers were negative at the time of diagnosis [44].

Patients should be observed for up to 10 years, for late recurrences, although they are rare.

6.11. Prognosis

- The prognosis of OGCT is excellent, as most cases are benign. When malignant they are very aggressive, but the prognosis is still good provided it is treated without delay with combination chemotherapy [8].
- Most patients with mature teratomas show long survival times.
- The prognosis of immature teratomas is governed by grade and stage. Stage 1, grade 1 have 100% survival rate, whereas stage III, grade 1 have only a 50% chance of survival.
- The survival rates for dysgerminomas presenting at early and advanced stages are 95 and >80%, respectively. In dysgerminoma stage 1a tumor after unilateral salpingo-oophorectomy as a fertility preserving surgery has a relapse rate ranging from 10 to 20%; the overall survival rate is 90–100% [45]. Patients who suffer relapses and undergo chemotherapy; the survival rate for such patients is greater than 90%.
- Endodermal sinus tumors of the ovary are particularly aggressive. The survival rates for stage I and II ESTs are reported to be 60–100%, whereas for those with stage III or IV disease the prognosis is less favorable (50–75%).
- Survival rates for embryonal carcinoma are slightly higher than those for ESTs.
- Prognosis is better for gestational choriocarcinoma than nongestational carcinoma.
- For mixed GCT, size and histology are the major factors determining prognosis for patients. Prognosis is poor for patients with large tumors when more than one-third of the tumor is composed of endodermal sinus elements, grade 3 immature teratoma or choriocarcinoma. When the tumor is smaller than 10 cm in diameter, the prognosis is good regardless of the composition of the tumor [46].
- Data from the Surveillance, Epidemiology and End Results program (1978–2010), investigators found a 97%, 5-year cause specific survival in those with ovarian dysgerminoma compared with a 92% for those with nondysgerminoma. Significant prognostic factors included age older than 40 years at diagnosis and metastatic disease. A second cancer occurred in 10% of all patients who survived 10 years and had received radiotherapy compared to 2% of those who had not received radiation treatment [47].

7. Dysgerminoma

The most commonly occurring malignant GCT is dysgerminoma, which accounts for approximately 2% of all ovarian cancers. It is the most common ovarian germ cell tumor coexisting with pregnancy, and constitutes 25–35% of all reported ovarian cancers. Mostly, it is diagnosed at an early stage, when disease is still confined to the ovary.

7.1. Etiology

The exact etiology of dysgerminomas is not identified, though recent molecular studies have implicated loss of function with potential tumor suppressor gene *TRC8/RNF139* as a possible etiology [48]. Cytogenetics reveals 12p abnormalities in 81% of cases [9].

7.2. Pathology

Dysgerminomas are mostly unilateral (15% of dysgerminomas are bilateral), solid, nodular. They have a smooth, bosselated (knobby) external surface, is soft, fleshy, either cream-colored, gray, pink or tan when cut. Hemorrhage and necrosis is common, but less prominent than other malignant tumors.

Histological examination of dysgerminomas show a proliferation of epithelioid cells admixed with mature lymphocytes arranged in sheets or small clusters which are separated by thin, fibrous septae resembling alveoli. The neoplastic cells are large and have moderate to high nucleus-to-cytoplasm ratios. Other features are round nuclei; vesicular chromatin; prominent nucleoli; clear to eosinophilic cytoplasm rich in glycogen and lipid; and distinct cell borders (**Figure 1**) [49].

Multinucleated forms may be present. Mitotic activity may be significant and may vary greatly, even within the same tumor; atypical mitoses may be seen. Noncaseating granulomas, syncytiotrophoblast-like giant cells and germinal center formation are not uncommon. Additionally, foci of hemorrhage, necrosis, and small microcalcifications may also be identified [49, 50].

The neoplastic cells of dysgerminomas express placental alkaline phosphatase (PLAP), CD117 (c-*kit*), OCT 3/4, SALL4, and, variably, cytokeratin [49]. Positive stain for OCT4 (strong nuclear staining) in 90%+ cells is seen.

They do not express epithelial membrane antigen (EMA), S100 protein, CD45 (LCA), or alpha-fetoprotein (AFP) [49]. Syncytiotrophoblast-like giant cells are the source of beta-hCG production. A negative stain for CK7, CK20, HMW keratin, CD30 and vimentin is also found [51].

7.3. Imaging in dysgerminomas

In dysgerminoma, characteristic imaging findings include multilobulated solid masses with prominent fibrovascular septa. The anechoic, low-signal-intensity, or low-attenuation

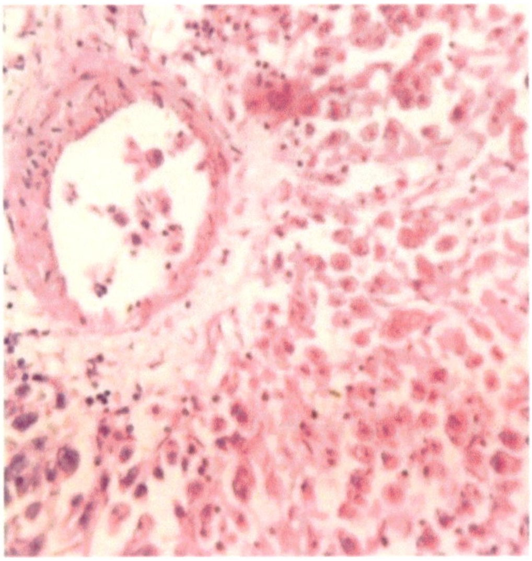

Figure 1. Dysgerminoma: Microsection showing tumor cells with vesicular nuclei. Fibrous septa showing lymphocytic infiltrate (400×, H&E stain). (With permission from [21]).

area of the tumor represents necrosis and hemorrhage. Lobules are richly vascularized at color/power Doppler examination which show prominent arterial flow within the fibro vascular septa with a resistive index value ranging from 0.44 to 0.70 [52]. On MRI, dysgerminomas are often seen divided into lobules by septa. Reported signal characteristics are hypointense or isointense septae on T2 weighted images. In T1 C+ (Gd) weighted images, the septae often show marked enhancement.

8. Teratoma

They represent 20% of all ovarian tumors, 75%, occur in first two decades of life, 12–15% are bilateral and 60–70% are diagnosed in stage 1.

Teratomas range from benign, well-differentiated (mature) cystic lesions to those that are solid and malignant (immature). Additionally, teratomas may be monodermal and highly specialized (struma ovarii, carcinoid). Rarely, in some mature teratomas containing certain elements (most commonly squamous components) undergo malignant transformation.

8.1. Mature cystic teratoma

Ovarian mature cystic teratomas, also called dermoid cysts, are the most common germ cell tumor, accounting for up to 70% of benign ovarian masses in the reproductive years and 20% in postmenopausal women [53, 54]. They maintain rather orderly arrangements, with well-differentiated ectodermal and mesodermal tissues surrounding endodermal components, resembling any tissue of the body. Examples include hair, teeth, fat, skin, muscle, and endocrine tissue (**Figure 2**).

Monodermal teratoma comprise of mainly one tissue element. For example, the most common type of monodermal teratoma, Struma ovarii, is comprised of at least 50% mature thyroid tissue (**Figures 3** and **4**). Argentaffin cells in dermoid cysts are usually the site of origin for ovarian carcinoid tumor, although this is rare (**Figure 5**).

Tumor markers-Mature teratomas rarely produce alpha feto protein and CA125.Elevated AFP and HCG levels may be indicative of malignancy.

8.1.1. Imaging

In mature cystic teratoma, transvaginal ultrasound scan (TVS) has 85–98% accuracy [55, 56]. Sonographic features includes: diffusely or partially echogenic mass with posterior sound attenuation owing to sebaceous material and hair within the cyst cavity, an echogenic interface at the edge of mass that obscures deep structures: the tip of the iceberg sign, mural hyperechoic Rokitansky nodule: dermoid plug, echogenic shadowing, calcific or dental

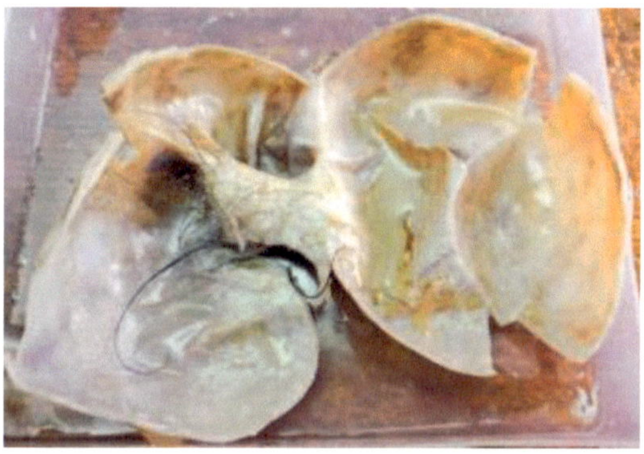

Figure 2. Dermoid cyst: cut section of dermoid cyst of ovary showing hairs and pultaceous material.

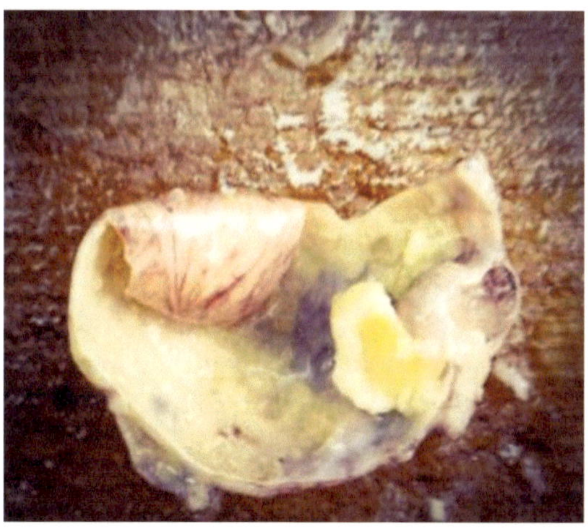

Figure 3. Struma ovarii: cut section of ovary containing pultaceous material along with gray white nodule measuring 2.5 × 2 cm.

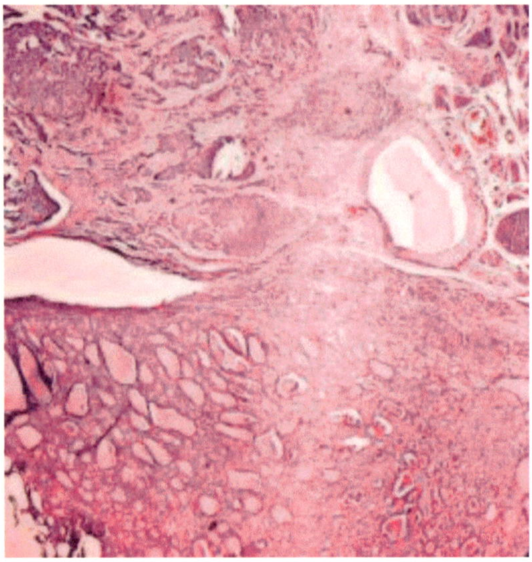

Figure 4. Struma ovarii: microsection showing thyroid tubules containing colloid in lower part of image. Upper part shows carcinoid element in which tumor cells are arranged in nests (4× H&E).

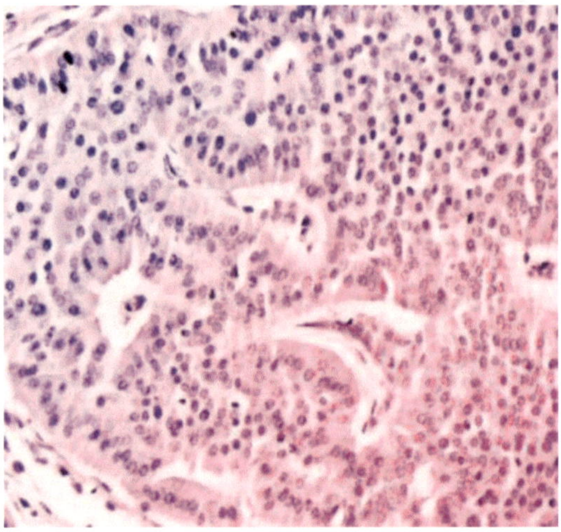

Figure 5. Carcinoid tumor: cells arranged in parallel ribbon like manner. Nuclei have characteristic salt and pepper like chromatin (40× H&E).

(tooth) components, the presence of fluid levels, multiple thin echogenic bands caused by the hair in the cyst cavity: the dot-dash pattern. In color Doppler, no internal vascularity is seen [57].

Further workup is required if internal vascularity is found to exclude a malignant lesion. When ruptured, the characteristic hypoattenuating fatty fluid can be found in antidependant pockets, typically below the right hemidiaphragm, a pathognomonic finding [58].

MR imaging is reported to have 99% accuracy. The sebaceous component of dermoid cysts has very high signal intensity on T1-weighted images similar to that of retroperitoneal fat. The signal intensity of the sebaceous component on T2-weighted images is variable, usually near that of fat [59].

8.1.2. Histology

Cyst cavity is often lined with keratinized squamous epithelium and usually contains abundant sebaceous and sweat glands (**Figure 6**). There is usually a raised protuberance projecting into the cyst cavity known as the Rokitansky nodule. Most of the hair typically arises from this protuberance. When bone or teeth are present, they tend to be located within this nodule. Occasionally, the cyst wall is lined with bronchial or gastrointestinal epithelium. Foreign body giant cell reactions may be seen in various parts of the tumor and may, in the case of intraperitoneal teratomas, lead to formation of extensive adhesions if the tumor contents are spilled. Ectodermal tissue may include brain, glia, neural tissue, retina, choroids, and ganglia. Mesodermal tissue is represented by bone, cartilage, smooth muscle, and fibrous tissue (**Figure 7**) [60].

8.1.3. Complications in teratoma

Torsion is the most significant cause of morbidity, occurring in 3–11% of cases [61, 62]. Rupture may occur suddenly in 2.5% [63] leading to shock or hemorrhage with acute chemical peritonitis. Chronic leakage also may occur, with resultant granulomatous peritonitis. Infection is uncommon and occurs in less than 1–2% of cases [63].

Malignant transformation: seen in 1–2%, usually into squamous cell carcinoma [64, 65].

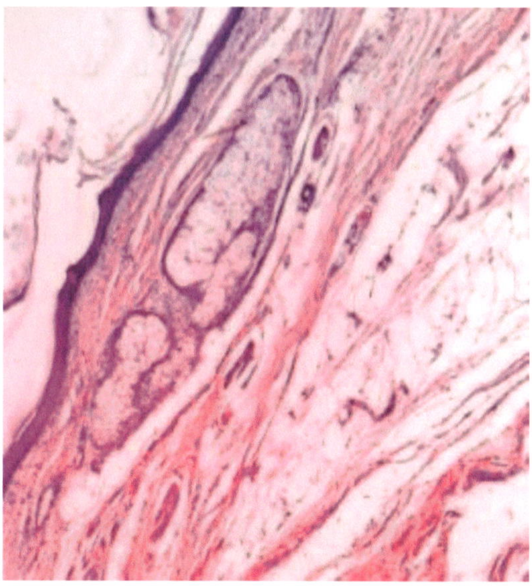

Figure 6. Mature cystic teratoma: microsection showing cystic lining with underlying sebaceous glands (40× H&E).

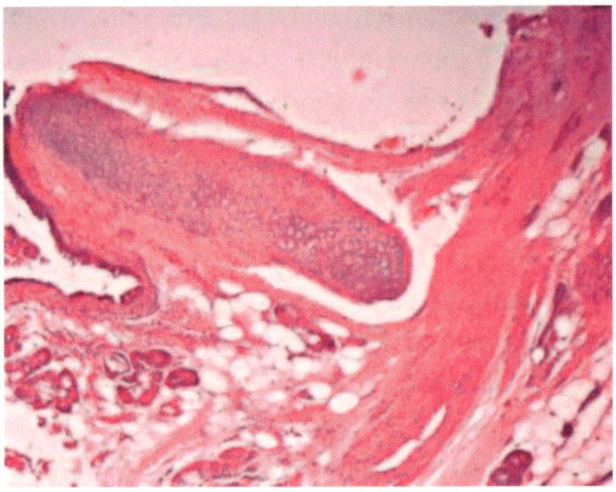

Figure 7. Dermoid cyst: microsection showing cartilaginous element (10× H&E).

In less than 1% autoimmune hemolytic anemia has been associated with mature cystic teratomas [66, 67]. Recently recognized encephalitis associated with antibodies against the *N*-methyl-D-aspartate receptor (NMDAR) is associated with ovarian mature teratomas. Substantial recovery is usually seen with tumor resection and immunotherapy [68].

8.1.4. Treatment

Mature ovarian teratomas are slow growing (1–2 mm a year) and, therefore, some advocate non-surgical management. Larger lesions are often surgically removed. Many recommend annual follow-up for lesions <7 cm to monitor growth, beyond which resection is advised. Mature cystic teratomas of the ovaries may be removed by simple cystectomy rather than salpingo-oophorectomy.

Although malignant degeneration is quite rare, the cyst should be removed in its entirety, and if immature elements are found, the patient should undergo a standard staging procedure.

Spillage is associated with increased risk of chemical peritonitis (estimated incidence of 0.2%) and increased risk of adhesion formation. The risks of recurrence (4%), as well as malignant degeneration (0.2–2%), should be discussed.

8.2. Immature teratoma

Immature cystic teratomas are rare (<3%) and usually occur in the postmenopausal age group [69]. Teratomas, specifically solid teratomas, are essentially devoid of organization. Immature teratomas account for approximately 20% of all malignant GCT. Immature teratomas are solid tumors containing immature or embryonal tissues (**Figure 8**). It is found either in pure form or as a component of a mixed germ cell tumor.

Immature neuroepithelium is the predominant immature tissue found. Grade is based upon the proportion of tissue containing immature neural elements and is considered an important prognostic factor that predicts extra ovarian spread and overall survival. They are classified as Grade I, II, or III if they have 0 or 1, 3 or less, or 4 or more low-power fields (x-40) containing immature neuroepithelium per slide, respectively [50].

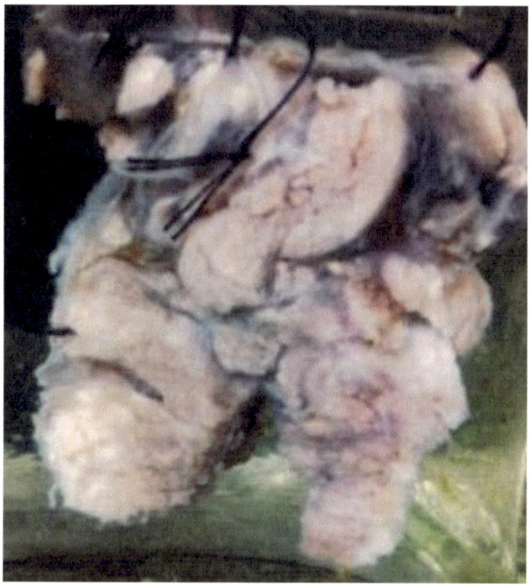

Figure 8. Immature teratoma of ovary: Irregular, partially encapsulated, solid tumor measuring 9 × 6 × 4 cm. Cut surface is grayish white with areas of hemorrhage and foci of necrosis.

8.2.1. Imaging

Immature teratomas have prominent solid components and may demonstrate internal necrosis or hemorrhage. Mature tissue elements similar to those seen in mature cystic teratoma are invariably present. Radiologic examination reveals a large, complex mass with cystic, solid components, and scattered calcifications; in contrast, calcification in mature teratomas is localized to mural nodules. Small foci of fat are also seen in immature teratomas. These tumors grow rapidly and frequently demonstrate perforation of the capsule. The tumor capsule is not always well defined.

8.2.2. Management of immature teratoma

Fertility-sparing surgery should be offered when detected during pregnancy with surgical staging. Thus unilateral salpingo-oophorectomy with preservation of contralateral ovary with uterus is the appropriate treatment in most cases. If metastatic disease is found during surgery, cytoreductive surgery is recommended. Stage 1a/G1 does not require adjunct treatment and can be observed. Chemotherapy is recommended when extra-ovarian disease exists, stage I grade 2–3. BEP is the most commonly used combination every 3 weeks for 3–4 courses.

8.2.3. Prognosis

The prognosis of immature teratomas is governed by grade and stage. Cases of grade 1 in stage I might have up to a 94% survival rate, whereas cases of grade 2 or 3 in stage I might drop to an 82% chance of survival. Grade also contributes to the recurrence rate, with higher grades having a higher recurrence rate [70, 71].

9. Endodermal sinus tumor or yolk sac tumor

Endodermal sinus tumor (EST), also known as yolk sac tumor, is a rare malignant ovarian tumor that usually occurs in the second decade of life. The tumor manifests as a large, complex pelvic mass that extends into the abdomen and contains both solid and cystic components. The cystic areas are composed of epithelial line cysts produced by the tumor or of co-existing mature teratomas. These tumors grow rapidly and have a poor prognosis. Affected patients have an elevated serum α-fetoprotein level, alpha 1 antitrypsin.

Gross examination of EST demonstrates smooth, glistening, hemorrhagic, and necrotic surfaces. Histology reveals a wide range of patterns (microcystic endodermal sinus, solid, alveolar-glandular, papillary, macrocystic, hepatoid, and primitive endodermal). On microscopic examination, it contains Schiller-Duval bodies (central capillary surrounded by simple papillae) and eosinophilic globules containing AFP (**Figure 9**). Intracellular and extracellular hyaline droplets (periodic acid-Schiff positive) are also seen in EST.

When diagnosed during pregnancy, it is often possible to continue the pregnancy after surgical staging and tumor debulking. For metastatic disease, the principles of cytoreductive surgery also apply, and the goal is the resection of all lesions to a minimal residual volume.

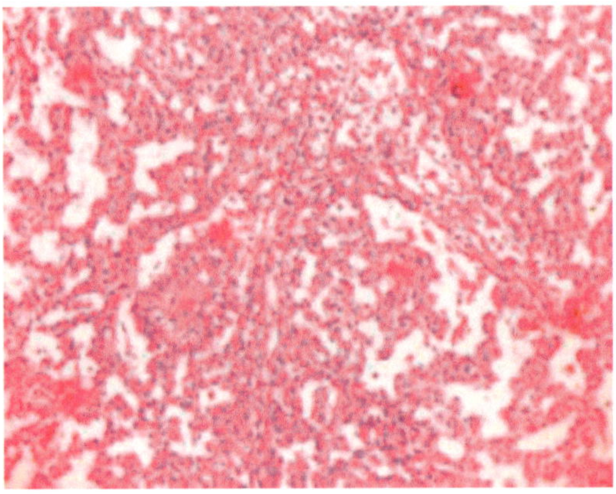

Figure 9. Yolk sac tumor: microsection showing Schiller-Duval bodies (40× H&E).

10. Non-gestational choriocarcinoma

In reproductive age group, the symptoms could resemble pregnancy with amenorrhoea and positive urine pregnancy test. The predominant presenting symptoms are lower abdominal pain, genital bleeding, amenorrhea, nausea and vomiting because of high levels of hCG. Choriocarcinoma is often diagnosed by finding an elevated hCG level in association with metastatic lesion detected radiographically. The levels of serum/urine beta hCG are good tumor marker for the progression or remission of disease. Paternal contribution present in the genome of the tumor is necessary to differentiate gestational from nongestational tumors. Serum β2 microglobulin may be used as a marker for non-gestational choriocarcinoma, though the cause of β2 microglobulin expression in non-gestational choriocarcinoma is unknown [72].

11. Pure embryonal carcinoma

It is rare in the ovary, may secrete estrogen, with patient exhibiting symptoms and signs of precocious puberty or irregular vaginal bleeding. Embryonal cell carcinoma has more nuclear hyperchromasia and nuclear pleomorphism, amphophilic cytoplasm, high mitotic index, and necrosis. Often, a glandular or papillary architecture is present. The cells of embryonal carcinoma express CD30 and cytokeratin (strong, diffuse), whereas those of dysgerminoma do not.

12. Mixed germ cell tumors

These are rare germ cell tumors. A mixture of dysgerminoma and endodermal sinus tumor is the most common combination accounting for one-third of mixed germ cell tumors [73]. Combination of embryonal carcinoma and choriocarcinoma is very rare. The prognosis of patients with a mixed MGCT usually reflects that of its most malignant component. Therefore, it is important to sample these tumors extensively, particularly areas with different gross appearance. One section per every centimeter in tumor diameter is recommended [74].

Acknowledgements

We acknowledge the contribution made by Dr. Namrata, Head of Pathology Deptt. Hindu Rao Hospital & NDMC Medical College for providing photographs for Figures 2-9.

Author details

Mamta Gupta* and Vandana Saini

*Address all correspondence to: hodgynaehrh@gmail.com

Hindu Rao Hospital & NDMC Medical College, New Delhi, India

References

[1] De Felici M 2013 Origin, migration, and proliferation of human primordial germ cells. In: Coticchio G, Albertinit DF, De Santis L (eds) Oogenesis. London: Springer; Ch. 2. pp. 19-37. DOI 10.1007/978-0-85729-826-3_2

[2] Schmoll HJ. Extragonadal germ cell tumors. Annals of Oncology. 2002;**13**(Suppl. 14):265-272

[3] Low JJH, Ilancheran A, Joseph SN. Malignant ovarian germ cell tumors. Best Practice and Research. Clinical Obstetrics & Gynaecology. 2012;**26**(3):347-355

[4] Smith HO, Berwick M, Verschraegen CF, Wiggins C, Lansing L, Muller CY, et al. Incidence and survival rates for female malignant germ cell tumors. Obstetrics and Gynecology. 2006;**107**(5):1075-1085

[5] Arora RS, Alston RD, Eden TO, Geraci M, Birch JM. Comparative incidence patterns and trends of gonadal and extragonadal germ cell tumors in England between 1979-2003. Cancer. 2012;**118**(17)4290-4297

[6] Abuzaid A, Nazer A, Alomar O, Azzam A, Al-Eid HS, Elhassan, TA et al. Incidence of Malignant Germ Cell Tumors (MOGCTs) in Saudi Arabia. Hematology/Oncology & Stem Cell Therapy. 2014;**7**(1):41-43

[7] Lee-Jones L. Ovary: Germ Cell Tumors. Atlas of Genetics and Cytogenetics in Oncology and Haematology. 2003-2008;**7**(4):282-288. http://atlasgeneticsoncology.org/Tumors/OvarianGermCellID5067.html

[8] Nogales F, Talerman A, Kubik-Huch RA, Tavassoli FA, Devouassoux-Shisheboran M. Germ cell tumours. In: Tavassoli FA, Deville P, editors. World Health Organization Classification of Tumours: Pathology and Genetics of Tumours of the Breast and Female Genital Organs. Lyon, France: IARC Press; 2003. pp. 163-175

[9] Cossu-Rocca P, Zhang S, Roth LM, Eble JN, Zheng W, Karim FW, et al. Chromosome 12p abnormalities in dysgerminoma of the ovary: A FISH analysis. Modern Pathology. 2006;**19**(4):611-615

[10] Kawauchi S, Liu XP, Kawasaki K, Hirakawa T, Amada S, Furuya T, et al. Significance of beta-catenin and pRB pathway components in malignant ovarian germ cell tumours: INK4A promoter CpG island methylation is associated with cell proliferation. The Journal of Pathology. 2004;**204**(3):268-276

[11] Giambartolomei C, Mueller CM, Greene MH, Korde LAA. Mini-review of familial ovarian germ cell tumors: An additional manifestation of the familial testicular germ cell tumor syndrome. Cancer Epidemiology. 2009;**33**(1):31-36

[12] Kraggerud SM, Hoei-Hansen CE, Alagaratnam S, Skotheim RI, Abeler VM, Rajpert-De Meyts E, et al. Molecular characteristics of malignant ovarian germ cell tumors and comparison with testicular counterparts: Implications for pathogenesis. Endocrine Reviews. 2013;**34**(3):339-376

[13] Cyriac S, Rajendranath R, Louis AR, Sagar TG. Familial germ cell tumor. Indian Journal of Human Genetics. 2012;**18**(1):119-121

[14] Prat J. FIGO committee on gynecologic oncology. FIGO's staging classification for cancer of ovary, fallopian tube and peritoneum: A bridged publication. Journal of Gynecologic Oncology. 2015;**26**(2):87-89

[15] Sayedur Rahman M, Al-Sibai MH, Rahman J. Ovarian carcinoma associate with pregnancy. A review of 9 cases. Acta Obstetricia et Gynecologica Scandinavica. 2002;**81**:260-264

[16] Zhao XY, Huang HF, Lian LJ, Lang JH. Ovarian cancer in pregnancy: A clinicopathologic analysis of 22 cases and review of the literature. International Journal of Gynecological Cancer. 2006;**16**:8-15

[17] Agarwal N, Parul, Kriplani A, Bhatla N, Gupta A. Management and outcome of pregnancies complicated with adnexal masses. Archives of Gynecology and Obstetrics. 2003;**267**(3):148-152

[18] Hopkins MP, Duchon MA. Adnexal surgery in pregnancy. The Journal of Reproductive Medicine. 1986;**31**:1035-1037

[19] Sunanda N, Akhila MV. Ovarian tumours associated with pregnancy: A five year retrospective study in a tertiary care hospital. International Journal of Reproduction, Contraception, Obstetrics and Gynecology. 2015;**4**(6):1965-1969

[20] Nick AM, Schmeler K. Adnexal masses in pregnancy. Perinatology. 2010;**2**:13-21

[21] Gupta M, Jindal R, Saini V. An incidental finding of bilateral dysgerminoma during cesarean section: Dilemmas in management. Journal of Clinical and Diagnostic Research. 2016;**10**(8):QD04-QD05

[22] Jain M, Budhwani C, Jain AK, Hazari RA. Pregnancy with ovarian dysgerminoma: An unusual diagnosis. Journal of Dental and Medical Sciences. 2013;**11**(5):53-57

[23] Hussain F. In: Huh WK, editor. Gynecologic Tumor Markers Overview. Medscape; 2015

[24] Kawai M, Kano T, Kikkawa F, Morikawa Y, Oguchi H, Nakashima N, et al. Seven tumor markers in benign and malignant germ cell tumors of the ovary. Gynecologic Oncology. 1992;**45**(3):248-253

[25] Behtash N, Karimi Zarchi M, Modares Gilani M, Ghaemmaghami F, Mousavi A, Ghotbizadeh F. Ovarian carcinoma associated with pregnancy: A clinicopathologic analysis of 23 cases and review of the literature. BMC Pregnancy and Childbirth. 2008;**20**(8):3. DOI: 10.1186/1471-2393-8-3

[26] Chiou SY, Lev-Toaff AS, Masuda E, Feld RI, Bergin D. Adnexal torsion: New clinical and imaging observations by sonography, computed tomography, and magnetic resonance imaging. Journal of Ultrasound in Medicine. 2007;**26**(10):1289-1301 PMID: 17901133

[27] Yen CF, Lin SL, Murk W, Wang CJ, Lee CL, Soong YK, et al. Risk analysis of torsion and malignancy for adnexal masses during pregnancy. Fertility and Sterility. 2009;**91**(5):1895-1902

[28] Karlen JR, Akbari A, Cook WA. Dysgerminoma associated with pregnancy. Obstetrics and Gynecology. 1979;**53**(3):330-335

[29] Zanetta G, Mariani E, Lissoni A, Ceruti P, Trio D, Strobelt N, Mariani S. A Prospective study of the role of ultrasound in the management of adnexal masses in pregnancy. BJOG: An International Journal of Obstetrics & Gynaecology. 2003;**110**(6):578-583

[30] Bernhard LM, Klebba PK, Gray DL, Mutch DG. Predictors of persistence of adnexal masses in pregnancy. Obstetrics and Gynecology. 1999;**93**(4):585-589

[31] Schmeler KM, Mayo-Smith WW, Peipert JF, Weitzen S, Manuel MD, Gordinier ME. Adnexal masses in pregnancy: Surgery compared with observation. Obstetrics and Gynecology. 2005;**105**(5 Pt 1):1098-1103

[32] Kwon YS, Mok JE, Lim KT, Lee IH, Kim TJ, Lee KH, Shim JU. Ovarian cancer during pregnancy: Clinical and pregnancy outcome. Journal of Korean Medical Science. 2010;**25**(2):230-234

[33] Horowitz NS. Management of adnexal masses in pregnancy. Clinical Obstetrics and Gynecology. 2011;**54**(4):519-527

[34] Zanotti KS, Belinson JL, Kennedy AW. Treatment of gynecologic cancers in pregnancy. Seminars in Oncology. 2000;**27**:686-698

[35] Partridge EE, Phillips JL, Menck HR. The National Cancer Data Base report on ovarian cancer treatment in United States hospitals. Cancer. 1996;**78**:2236-2246

[36] Cavaco-Gomes J, Moreira CJ, Rocha A, Mota R, Paiva V, Costa A. Investigation and management of adnexal masses in pregnancy. Scientifica. 2016;**2016**:3012802. DOI: 10.1155/2016/3012802

[37] Wang PH, Chang WH, Cheng MH, Horng HC. Management of adnexal masses during pregnancy. The Journal of Obstetrics and Gynaecology Research. 2009;**35**(3):597-598

[38] Whitecar MP, Turner S, Higby MK. Adnexal masses in pregnancy: A review of 130 cases undergoing surgical management. American Journal of Obstetrics and Gynecology. 1999;**181**:19-24

[39] Usui R, Minakami H, Kosuge S, Iwasaki R, Ohwada M, Sato I. A retrospective survey of clinical, pathologic, and prognostic features of adnexal masses operated on during pregnancy. The Journal of Obstetrics and Gynaecology Research. 2000;**26**(2):89-93

[40] Mazze RI, Kallén B. Reproductive outcome after anesthesia and operation during pregnancy: A registry study of 5405 cases. American Journal of Obstetrics and Gynecology. 1989;**161**(5):1178-1185

[41] Williams S, Blessing JA, Liao SY, Ball H, Hanjani P. Adjuvant therapy of ovarian germ cell tumors with cisplatin, etoposide, and bleomycin: a trial of the Gynecologic Oncology Group. Journal of Clinical Oncology. 1994 Apr;**12**(4):701-706

[42] Jewell EL. Germ Cell Tumor Treatment Protocols. In: Sonoda Y, editor. Medscape; 2015. Available at: https://emedicine.medscape.com/article/2156882-overview

[43] Hasdemir PS, Guvenal T, Meneske S, Solmaz U, Kandiloglu AR, Koyuncu FM, et al. Ovarian immature teratoma detected during pregnancy. Medical Science and Discovery. 2016;**3**(1):1-6

[44] Michener CM, Wu AY. Ovarian Dysgerminomas Follow-Up. In: Huh WK, editor. Medscape; 2015. Available at: https://emedicine.medscape.com/article/253701-followup

[45] Pectasides D, Pectasides E, Kassanos D. Germ cell tumors of the ovary. Cancer Treatment Reviews. 2008;**34**(5):427-441

[46] Murugaesu N, Schmid P, Dancey G, et al. Malignant ovarian germ cell tumors: Identification of novel prognostic markers and long-term outcome after multimodality treatment. Journal of Clinical Oncology. 2006;**24**(30):4862-4866

[47] Solheim O, Gershenson DM, Trope CG, Rokkones E, Sun CC, Weedon-Fekjaer H, et al. Prognostic factors in malignant ovarian germ cell tumours (the surveillance, epidemiology and end results experience 1978-2010). European Journal of Cancer. 2014;**50**(11):1942-1950

[48] Gimelli S, Beri S, Drabkin HA, Gambini C, Gregorio A, Fiorio P, et al. The tumor suppressor gene TRC8/RNF139 is disrupted by a constitutional balanced translocation t(8;22)(q24.13;q11.21) in a young girl with dysgerminoma. Molecular Cancer. 2009;**8**:52

[49] Hazard FKG. Ovarian Dysgerminomas Pathology Overview of Ovarian Dysgerminomas. Masand R. Medscape; 2015 available at https://emedicine.medscape.com/article/1951026-overview

[50] Sharma I, Chaliha T. Histopathological patterns of germ cell tumours of ovary in a tertiary level hospital. International Journal of Pharmaceutical Science Inventions. 2014;**3**(10):14-24

[51] Ehdaivand S. Ovary Tumor, Germ Cell Tumors, Dysgerminoma. 2016. Pathology outlines.com

[52] Kim HS, Kang BS. Ovarian dysgerminoma: Color Doppler ultrasonographic findings and comparison with CT and MR imaging findings. Journal of Ultrasound in Medicine. 1995;**14**:843-848

[53] Pfeifer SM, Gosman GG. Evaluation of adnexal masses in adolescents. Pediatric Clinics of North America. 1999;**46**(3):573-592

[54] Canis M, Mage G, Pouly JL, Wattiez A, Manhes H, Bruhat MA. Laparoscopic diagnosis of adnexal cystic masses: A 12-year experience with long-term follow-up. Obstetrics & Gynecology. 1994;**83**(5):707-712 Part 1

[55] Mais V, Guerriero S, Ajossa S, Angiolucci M, Paoletti AM, Melis GB. Transvaginal ultrasonography in the diagnosis of cystic teratoma. Obstetrics and Gynecology. 1995;**85**(1):48-52

[56] Patel MD, Feldstein VA, Lipson SD, Chen DC, Filly RA. Cystic teratomas of the ovary: Diagnostic value of sonography. AJR. American Journal of Roentgenology. 1998;**171**:1061-1065

[57] Kite L, Uppal T. Ultrasound of ovarian dermoids—Sonographic findings of a dermoid cyst in a 41-year-old woman with an elevated serum hCG. Australasian Journal of Ultrasound in Medicine. 2011;**14**(3):19-21

[58] Fibus TF. Intraperitoneal rupture of a benign cystic ovarian teratoma: Findings at CT and MR imaging. AJR. American Journal of Roentgenology. 2000;**174**(1):261-262

[59] Scoutt LM, McCarthy SM, Lange R, Bourque A, Schwartz PE. MR evaluation of clinically suspected adnexal masses. Journal of Computer Assisted Tomography. 1994;**18**(4):609-618

[60] Talerman A. Germ cell tumors of the ovary. In: Kurman RJ, editor. Blaustein's Pathology of the Female Genital Tract. 5th ed. New York, NY: Springer-Verlag; 2002 Chap. 20

[61] Comerci JT Jr, Licciardi F, Bergh PA, Gregori C, Breen JL. Mature cystic teratoma: a clinicopathologic evaluation of 517 cases and review of the literature. Obstetrics and Gynecology. 1994;**84**(1):22-28

[62] Benjapibal M, Boriboonhirunsarn D, Suphanit I, Sangkarat S. Benign cystic teratoma of the ovary: A review of 608 patients. Journal of The Medical Association of Thailand. 2000;**83**(9):1016-1020

[63] Ayhan A, Bukulmez O, Genc C, Karamursel BS, Ayhan A. Mature cystic teratomas of the ovary: Case series from one institution over 34 years. European Journal of Obstetrics, Gynecology, and Reproductive Biology. 2000;**88**(2):153-157

[64] Hosokawa T, Sato Y, Seki T, Maebara M, Ito K, Kuribayashi S. Malignant transformation of a mature cystic teratoma of the ovary with rupture. Japanese Journal of Radiology. 2010;**28**(5):372-375

[65] Dos Santos L, Mok E, Iasonos A, et al. Squamous cell carcinoma arising in mature cystic teratoma of the ovary: A case series and review of the literature. Gynecologic Oncology. 2007;**105**(2):321-324

[66] Buchwalter CL, Miller D, Jenison EL. Hemolytic anemia and benign pelvic tumors. A case report. The Journal of Reproductive Medicine. 2001;**46**(4):401-404

[67] Kim I, Lee JY, Kwon JH, et al. A case of autoimmune hemolytic anemia associated with an ovarian teratoma. Journal of Korean Medical Science. 2006;**21**(2):365-367

[68] Dalmau J, Lancaster E, Martinez-Hernandez E, Rosenfeld MR, Balice-Gordon R. Clinical experience and laboratory investigations in patients with anti-NMDAR encephalitis. Lancet Neurology. 2011;**10**(1):63-74

[69] Christopherson WA, Councell RB. Malignant degeneration of amatureovarian teratoma. International Journal of Gynecology & Obstetrics. 1989;**30**(4):379-384

[70] O'Connor DM, Norris HJ. The influence of grade on the outcome of stage I ovarian immature (malignant) teratomas and the reproducibility of grading. International Journal of Gynecological Pathology. 1994;**13**:283-289

[71] Norris HJ, Zirkin HJ, Benson WL. Immature (malignant) teratoma of the ovary: A clinical and pathologic study of 58 cases. Cancer. 1976;**37**:2359-2372

[72] Hayashi S, Abe Y, Tomita S, Nakanishi Y, Miwa S, Nakajima T, et al. Primary non-gestational pure choriocarcinoma arising in the ovary: A case report and literature review. Oncology Letters. 2015;**9**(5):2109-2111

[73] Kurman RJ, Norris HJ. Embryonal carcinoma of the ovary: A clinicopathological entity distinct from endodermal sinus tumour resembling embryonal carcinoma of adult testes. Cancer. 1976;**38**(6):2420-2433

[74] Prat J. Ovarian Germ Cell Tumors in Pathology of the Female Reproductive Tract. 2015. https://clinicalgate.com/ovarian-germ-cell-tumors/